WEAPONS OF FITNESS

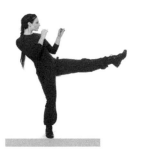

WEAPONS
OF FITNESS

The Women's Ultimate Guide to Fitness,
Self-Defense, and Empowerment

AVITAL ZEISLER

AVERY
A member of Penguin Group (USA)
New York

Published by the Penguin Group
Penguin Group (USA) LLC
375 Hudson Street
New York, New York 10014

USA • Canada • UK • Ireland • Australia
New Zealand • India • South Africa • China

penguin.com
A Penguin Random House Company

Most Avery books are available at special quantity discounts for bulk purchase for sales promotions, premiums, fund-raising, and educational needs. Special books or book excerpts also can be created to fit specific needs. For details, write Special.Markets@us.penguingroup.com

ISBN: 978-1-58333-569-7

Printed in the United States of America
1   3   5   7   9   10   8   6   4   2

BOOK DESIGN BY TANYA MAIBORODA

I dedicate this book to every woman,
with the hopes that, together,
we can train and create a life we love,
armed with the knowledge to protect ourselves
both physically and mentally.

CONTENTS

PART 3
HITTING YOUR TARGETS

PART 4
PROTECTING YOUR LIFE

ACKNOWLEDGMENTS

To my family, who built the nest, told me I had the wings to fly, and trusted that I could achieve my dreams—I would not be who I am if not for your love and support. For all who inspired me throughout this journey, I offer you my gratitude and respect. I recall every moment of support vividly, and I want to thank those who believed in me along the way—your generosity of spirit has helped me find the place where I can share this method with the world. To my literary agent, Joy Tutela, and my editors at Penguin, Megan Newman and Gigi Campo, for seeing this vision through—I could not have done this without you. To the one man who endured the impact of every combative featured in this book—thank you, George, for your physical and emotional generosity. To Tammy, I am forever grateful for your unwavering support. To Richard and Amy, thank you for your support, guidance, and belief in the cause—from the outset. Moran Cerf, thank you for your time consulting with me on the neuroscience of our minds. Dax, thank you for being my rock. To every one of my students—I am honored and humbled by your achievements. All of you give me the extra strength to move forward, as you have all touched my spirit in a special and unique way.

FOREWORD

I had always subscribed to the belief that women were far more likely to be victimized by men because they were physically weaker and thus ill-equipped to defend themselves. This was nonsense that, I suppose, was further perpetuated by my love of movies—where, time and time again, I was offered examples of the classic "damsel in distress." It wasn't until I met Avital Zeisler and was introduced to her unique method of self-defense, the Soteria Method, that my perceptions were forever changed. There's no clearer way to say this (and I hope I don't lose anyone by speaking so technically), but Avital is a genuine badass. She emboldened me beyond my wildest expectations by teaching me simple mechanical techniques and combative wisdom that more than make up for any physical disadvantage. In short, she turned *me* into a badass. The Soteria Method is exclusively for the female defender and works for women of all ages and sizes. It helps you to build an effective and intuitive survival mindset that ensures your ability to use the concepts and strategies under pressure. Learning Avital's method has actually made me less paranoid and more confidently aware.

In addition to learning how to physically defend myself, I was surprised by my gains in mental acuity and my reduction of anxiety. Avital's Soteria Method gave me an increased level of confidence, which resonates in my daily life. It's also a serious workout. Avital's personal journey is intertwined in her method and profoundly illustrates how women can gain strength to overcome any attack, setback, or negative experience—and to live the best life possible.

Avital's story is a fascinating one. She is incredibly brave for sharing it. It is her personal experience of surviving a sexual assault and becoming such a highly respected self-defense instructor that gives the Soteria Method such strength, purity, and authenticity. Here, embedded in her ethos, you'll find a unique set of benefits for women of every age, state of mind, and physical capability.

I believe that every woman should know the Soteria Method. Life is too precious to not want to get the most out of it, so strive for happiness and solace. The physical and mental benefits of learning Avital's method will be apparent shortly after a commitment to her program. The empowerment that you feel will last a lifetime.

— A M A N D A   S E Y F R I E D

WEAPONS OF FITNESS

YOUR
MISSION

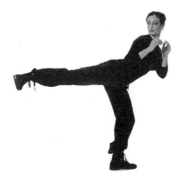

REDEFINING
SELF-DEFENSE FOR WOMEN

▼

I was told that I was too tall to be a classical ballerina. I was told that I had too much muscle in my calves to be a model. I was told that I didn't have a deep-enough six-pack when I participated in a fitness competition for athletic routines. My body never fit society's molds for the passions I wanted to pursue. Being judged on each and every physical attribute, rather than who I was as an individual, sometimes made me feel like a prisoner to my appearance. But deep inside, no matter what anyone said, I had a drive to find my place in the world, and a dream to nurture a creative outlet where I could express who I was and what happiness meant to me.

When I was young, I always considered happiness a given. I was totally immersed in the world of dance, got good grades, and maintained my focus on being the best dancer and student I could be. I felt invincible, safe, loved, supported, and cherished by my family and friends. I was completely unaware that bad things could happen to me. Even when a neighbor surprised me on my driveway by telling me that I was his "honey," all I had to do was tell my father. He immediately marched over to the neighbor's house and made sure that was the last time this neighbor came anywhere near me or our property, or the police would be called. Within this cocoon of security, I nourished my ambition.

When I was thirteen, I insisted that my mother take me to my first serious dance audition, and soon I moved away from home to attend a full-time ballet school. As the years passed, I competed in every dance competition that I could, and dieted until I had a model's measurements and became part of the fabulous fashion industry. Not content with success in dance and modeling, I also worked tirelessly in school to get the best marks possible, just in case I ever decided to become a doctor. I was ambitious and driven, but I was still a typical kid, juggling my grades and my passions with my life outside high school. And even after my neighbor's comment, I remained totally oblivious to potential danger.

Then, one time when I was walking home from my bus stop, I realized that a car was following me. I was scared, but I kept my cool and cut in between some houses to lose him. When I told my parents, my father immediately signed me up for a Krav Maga class. Krav Maga is the official self-defense system of the Israeli Defense Forces and has been adapted for use by elite combat units, secret service operatives, law enforcement, and the general public. I enrolled in a beginner class, learned the moves, and aced the test. The whole time, I was more concerned with getting a high mark on my final Krav Maga test than with actually contemplating the reasons for learning the moves and their effectiveness for real-life application.

DURING MY FIRST YEAR of college, I met a man. I was so taken with him. He said the right things, acted as if tending to my needs was his purpose in life, and spoke as if he supported each and every one of my dreams. As a naive young woman who believed I was in love, I bought it all! This was my first serious relationship, and it felt wonderful. Even as he became increasingly controlling and jealous, no one—not my parents, brothers, or friends—could tell me anything against him, because I wouldn't hear it.

I started spending more and more time with him at his place and envisioned a long future together. But then one night we got into an argument. I didn't want to do something sexual with him, and he was insisting. I refused, and he lost it.

Within seconds, he turned into a raging monster and lunged at me. I was in utter shock as he grabbed my hair and banged my head into the bathroom wall. Three times. Each time he asked me if I would give in and do what he wanted.

All I could do was think, "What is happening? How could he be doing this to me? Where did this violence come from? Why did my saying no to him result in this violence? What am I going to do?" These and millions of other thoughts ran through my mind. I had no idea how to get out of his hold of my hair, which was incredibly painful. He asked me again if I would do it, and I said no again. He whirled me around and started shoving my head toward the toilet bowl. I resisted, trying to keep my head out of the water, and then I decided to try to calm him down. I cried out that I would do what he wanted. He released my hair to let me up. I ran out of the bathroom and tried to run out of the bedroom, but he leaped after me and grabbed me. He swung to punch me, but I somehow blocked it, through natural reflexes (not training). Then he choked me around the neck. Somehow, with my minimal training, I was able to get out of the choke hold. Then he pinned me down and violently raped me.

I was in utter disbelief that this had happened to me—that someone who'd said that he loved and adored me could attack me so violently. I could not wrap my head around the implications of his attack—what it meant for me as a woman, what it made him as a man. I wondered how I could ever move on from the devastation I felt.

The physical damage was nothing compared to the emotional trauma, which would not go away. Every aspect of positivity and daily enjoyment in life had vanished. I felt nothing but negativity—toward everything and everyone. I had been so innocent, so sure of my own invincibility, and I'd felt so cherished by my family. But now I was damaged inside and out. I was a person who no longer had a direct line to her dreams and aspirations.

After a few days, I told my parents about what had happened. We decided that I needed to at least get a protection order against him. When we went to the police, they said he should be charged with both sexual and physical assault. He was arrested and charged. Every time I tried to pretend like it hadn't happened or to ignore my flashbacks, another meeting with the police or people from the Victim Services agency would remind me of the incident and the upcoming court case in which I would testify. I didn't want to serve as a witness, but I couldn't get over the fact that if I didn't, I would potentially be putting another woman's life at risk.

As I waited for the case to make its way through the court system, I learned more about sexual assault from the information provided by Victim Services and individual therapy. I'd thought that since I personally knew the man who had attacked me, it wasn't considered rape. I was shocked to learn that, according to the Bureau of Justice Statistics, 78 percent of female rape or sexual assault victims from 2005 to 2010 were assaulted by friends, acquaintances, family members, or intimate partners, while only 22 percent were attacked by strangers (per the Bureau of Justice Statistics 2013 report *Female Victims of Sexual Violence, 1994–2010*). I gained many other unwelcome insights like this as I tried to come to terms with my assault and how it had permanently changed me. One of the most difficult things to accept was that I was only one of thousands of women who have faced this—and worse.

As an athletic kid and teenager, I had always sought out some form of physical activity, whether for exercise or simply to put me in a good mood. But after the incident, nothing made me feel any sense of confidence, empowerment, or positivity. I tried dance classes, fitness classes, every activity I could think of. Soon it got to the point where I had to find a way to bring myself back to life.

I decided to take another self-defense class and reintroduced myself to Krav Maga, since my father still recommended it as an effective self-defense system. This time in class, I was actually able to learn the defenses against the attack that I had experienced. I learned how I could have fought back in the incident, and I practiced the moves over and over again. I gained confidence with each repetition.

I was amazed at the changes I felt. For the first time since the incident, I began to feel the sense of empowerment and confidence that I was so longing for. I kept on going back to the self-defense classes just to hold on to those positive feelings. I soon became addicted.

My transformation began with a search for empowerment, but it quickly became a more involved challenge of assessing how what I was being taught was applicable to women in particular. Basically, I wanted to find out if I, as a woman, could really defend myself against a much stronger and larger attacker. Since I'd experienced a violent sexual assault firsthand, I had a unique lens of reality that I used to assess the concepts and tactics that I was shown. I couldn't help but try to judge whether or not each tactic I was shown would work in a real-life situation.

From my experience, I knew that at the moment of the attack, I was feeling so many things, had so many thoughts, that I wasn't able to formulate a clear or quick response. In the moment, I was trying to simultaneously comprehend what was happening, overcome the pain and fear I felt at this sudden betrayal and attack, *and* formulate an escape plan. There was too much going on in my head, and I was ill prepared to defend myself. Knowing how my brain reacted in this situation informed my approach to learning self-defense techniques. I knew these factors had to be kept in mind when assessing the effectiveness of the self-defense techniques I was being shown.

So, whenever I was taught a new move in a training session, I would respectfully and quietly challenge the technique in my mind, rather than accept it at face value. I would picture myself back in the moment when I'd been attacked and ask myself, If I had known how to do this Backhand Hammer Fist, would it have helped me in that situation? Would I have been able to think of it in time for it to be helpful? I challenged each move in my mind and on the mat, and I tested or modified what I learned on my own after class. It even started to feel fun— becoming a new game of physical angles, leverages, body mechanics, and mindset boundary adjustments. I became fascinated with finding defensive tactics and solutions that did not rely on my size or strength.

As I immersed myself more and more into the world of self-defense, I had an epiphany. I realized that the perceived disadvantages of being a woman could actually work to the *advantage* of a female defender. Our smaller statures can be very misleading to a larger, stronger attacker. No matter how small we are, if we are well trained, we are still capable of exerting force toward targets. And on the psychological level, male attackers will perceive us as weaker and physically inferior. So if a woman is able to stay tactical while under attack, she'll have the element of surprise on her side.

I continued exploring why self-defense meant such different things for men and women, and revelation after revelation excited me and drove me to learn all I could about self-defense from a woman's perspective.

AFTER SOME BASIC self-defense training in my hometown of Toronto, I sought out more advanced classes and began to train in the United States. Then I was invited to attend a Krav Maga training session in Israel, and I jumped at the chance to learn about this powerful fighting style at its source. People told me that no woman had ever passed the full instructor course, and that since I was only twenty years old, I was still too new to the system to do so. But that challenge was all I needed to hear. I packed my bags with my brand-new Krav Maga equipment and joined thirty-five men from around the world in the instructor course.

In some of my previous training sessions, the male participants had been dismissive of me and didn't believe that I could hold my own against them. So it was no surprise when I encountered the same skepticism in this instructor course. One very vocal skeptic, in particular, chose to pick on me during the first week to try to show how much I didn't belong there. Then, one time, he made the mistake of trying to kick me, thinking I wouldn't know how to block it. I blocked it with my leg. His shin shattered. This story continues to circle back to me even now, years later. It was the moment that earned me the grudging respect of the other participants—and the reputation of being the "Canadian girl who could hold her own." I worked hard, trained harder, and passed the instructor course.

My time spent studying Krav Maga only reinforced my realization that self-defense is very different for men and women. Knowing Krav Maga as well as I did only made me want to learn more about other forms of self-defense. So I sought out opportunities to learn from as many military personnel, law enforcement officials, and security specialists from around the world as I could. This was the pivotal point when I committed myself to my mission of finding out what was real self-defense. I was able to use my own experience of a violent attack to zero in on effective self-defense techniques for women. I could still remember the sense of freezing in fear during my own attack, so each time I mastered a technique and mentally tested it against my attacker, I felt a sense of immense satisfaction and relief.

MY NEW QUEST had enabled me to shift from a negative mindset to a more workable one. I was functional, though I still wasn't happy or excited about life. I attended my college classes and listened to what my professors were saying, but I had a very hard time connecting with people. And whenever I could, I would head off for training sessions or go on trips to further my study. When I finally graduated from college, it was easy for me to make the decision to teach self-defense.

After years of studying and training, I finally felt like I could defend myself against an attack if I needed to. But I wanted every woman to have that sense of confidence. As my passion to show others what I had learned became more and more meaningful to me, I decided to make the big move to New York City to work as a hand-to-hand-combat consultant.

I continued to train and expand my network of security contacts, but I still couldn't pull myself from the state of being on emotional autopilot. I struggled to make it in New York as some of the friends and contacts I had trusted the most let me down. I felt completely lost. And it was during this moment, my lowest moment in New York, that my original question of defining real self-defense was finally answered.

At this juncture, I asked myself, "What's the point of learning all this self-defense if you can't be happy and live the most of every moment?" And then it clicked. For the first time I saw self-defense as more than just a means to defend my physical body against violence. I realized then that the definition of "self-defense" should be about attacking life, not letting it attack you. I wanted my self-defense training to protect my state of mind and my positive reactions to life. I wanted it to let me live life not in a constant state of fear, but to allow me to feel vulnerable sometimes, emotionally or otherwise, and to let my guard down so that I would be open to new experiences. I wanted to actually be present for the important moments, instead of constantly looking for an escape or keeping an eye out for threats. This is what I wanted self-defense to do for me, and this is what I realized it could mean for everyone.

I wanted my physical self-defense tactics to protect my life—not just my physical body, but the confidence and courage I needed in order to live a fully open, vulnerable life without having to constantly keep my guard up. In order to make sure my training could protect my life, I had to learn how to live. I had to put an end to the negativity I'd allowed myself to feel ever since my attack and to transition toward valuing and appreciating the life I had been given and the possibilities the future held. So, in my attempts to start living, I found myself training emotionally as much as I was physically and mentally in self-defense. I fought to begin each day in a positive way—even though it usually meant a couple of mental rounds in the emotional ring. As time passed, I began to feel things again and to open up a bit more.

The lesson I learned was this: I'd been labeled a victim, and I'd allowed that label to permeate my sense of self. But I had the power to stop living my life as a victim. I realized that all of my negativity was from the past and that, in fact, I was the only one keeping the past in the present. I learned how to live more in the moment and how to open up to protect the moments in life that I wanted to experience. I stopped worrying about things that were out of my control, and I finally felt that anything was possible.

It was with this profound new outlook that I decided to teach and develop my own way of self-defense for women. I began to test the emotional discoveries along with the physical and tactical discoveries of my evolving self-defense system with others. As I watched my female clients transform, I felt a resurgence of the confident me, the fearless me. It brought me back to life.

My assault had had a profound effect on me. It had brought negativity and fear into every aspect of my life. But against all odds, I had found a way to live with positivity and determination, and I couldn't wait to share these insights and discoveries with women everywhere. I had found my purpose and a new meaning in life: I was going to help women protect their dreams.

I became dedicated to finding the best physical and emotional tactics for women's self-defense, and when it all came together, I called it the Soteria Method. I picked the name Soteria, which is the name of the Greek goddess of safety, because it represents the essence of safety, protection, and preservation from harm. I consider all of us to be goddesses in our own right—with the ability to safeguard ourselves and our loved ones.

The Soteria Method is a guide to helping you find your inner goddess of safety. In *Weapons of Fitness*, my very first book, you will learn how to avoid or physically defend yourself against the threat or act of violence. Incidentally, you'll also find yourself sculpting a lean, strong physique with the *Weapons of Fitness* workouts. And most important, you will discover an inner empowerment that will enable you to emotionally let your guard down and begin to create and live a life that you love.

My clients come into my course for various reasons and, no matter who they are, leave the course feeling empowered, strengthened, and much more confident. My client Jessica shared with me that she had never before felt so capable of taking care of herself as she traveled to and from work. Another client, Carol, used her newfound sense of empowerment to take on more challenges in her professional life—and succeeded! A client who had been assaulted as a teenager explained that she finally, after so many years, began to feel like the person she'd been before her attack—and was able to move on with a profound sense of confidence. The Soteria Method can change your life!

My method is simple, effective, and retainable, and above all, it is customizable for who you are and what you want to achieve. On the physical level, you and everyone else who read this book will all learn the same approach to physical protection and fitness. But on an emotional level, your own experience of this book will be unique. It doesn't matter what your specific goals are—what matters is that you want to bring positive change into your life and that you are the architect of this change. You opened this book with the desire to make a difference in your life, and I promise you, no matter what inabilities or weaknesses you think you have, you are capable of great change and accomplishment.

This unique discovery, and ultimately transformation, comes from the development of the survival mindset for self-defense, which I will teach you and which will allow you to tap into the strong and confident side of your personality. The Soteria Method lets you maintain your femininity, both physically and mentally, while allowing you to hold your own against a larger and stronger attacker.

Many people cling to the misconception that a woman needs to be some type of military robot to be strong and capable of defending herself. You will learn this is not true. You do not need to compromise yourself or change who you are by adopting a cold heart or living your life in paranoia. Being in constant fear or limiting your daily activities is not a productive way to deal with the risk of violence. Arming yourself with practical violence-prevention tactics and self-defense knowledge through concepts and techniques is the best way to assure your safety— not to mention your day-to-day happiness. Though it is certainly true that any woman can find herself facing violence anywhere and anytime, there is no point to living in constant fear and having your quality of life compromised by the threat of violence or a violent act. Instead, once you learn my method, you will focus on being able to attack the life you want, while at the same time not letting life attack you.

The principles in this book have served me well whenever I've faced tough challenges or crushing moments of weakness. And as you learn these moves and internalize these principles, you'll find every bit of support that you need—because I am in this with you. Your ambitions, your drive, and your dreams are worth safeguarding, and I can show you how; because there really is a way of becoming your own warrior goddess—the protector of your life and future.

I once strove to meet society's standards of beauty as I dieted my way into becoming a model, but my body no longer holds the power to affect the way I feel based on measurements or comparison with ideals in the media. I refuse to succumb to the power of judgment, stereotype, or arbitrary definitions of beauty or femininity. My body is my weapon to create the life that I want, and I will train it, nourish it, preserve it, and honor it.

A REAL TRANSFORMATION

I've trained thousands of women in the principles and tactics that you'll soon learn, and in most cases I came up against the same initial feeling. Almost every single woman first thought that she wouldn't be able to successfully defend herself against a real physical threat. One woman thought she was too physically weak for her blows to be effective; another thought she wouldn't be able to respond quickly enough to neutralize the threat; another admitted that she would outright freeze and couldn't react at all. Regardless of their specific justifications, all these women had one thing in common: denial. Denial of the possibility that they might someday experience violence; denial that they might be able to fight back; denial that women can fight men and win.

Because of fear and a lack of confidence, many women minimize or disregard their responsibility toward ensuring their own safety and the safety of their loved ones. I have to admit that before my journey of self-defense training and self-discovery, I too subscribed to some of these common beliefs:

- This kind of thing won't happen to me. (Denial)
- I can rely on a man to protect me. (Shirking responsibility)
- I don't go anywhere dangerous, so it won't happen to me. (Compromising your own quality of life out of fear)
- Others will come to my rescue as long as I scream. (Shirking responsibility and wishful thinking)
- I'm not strong enough to defend myself against a male attacker, so what's the point of trying to fight back? (Victim mindset)

Let me be very clear here: If the worst should happen and you are attacked, there is no guarantee that anybody will be around or within earshot to help you. You are ultimately in control of your safety, and if you're trained in self-defense, you stand a real chance of successfully fighting off your attacker. Did you know that 86 percent of women who fight back survive a violent encounter? I mean it when I tell you that this workout could save your life.

Let me give you a sample scenario. Let's say that you're walking home from work. You round the corner of a building and find yourself in a dimly lit space with no one else around. A stranger confronts you. When he grabs your arm, what should you do first? You probably don't know, and that's fine. This book will teach you the best type of release to use in this situation.

Fast-forward a couple of weeks in which you've been following the workouts in this book carefully and visualizing real-world applications of each move. Picture yourself standing on a deserted subway platform. A man approaches you and seems aggressive. Things escalate, and before you know it, he's trying to knock you down. However, because of your training, you don't panic and you're able to fight him off with an elbow combative. Just for clarification, a combative is any forceful movement involving a surface area on your body making direct contact with an intended target on another person.

He staggers in confusion, giving you a few seconds to act, and you take the opportunity to run down the platform to the station booth, where you're safe.

You may still be in denial about your chances of facing a real physical threat like the ones I've mentioned above, but the fact of the matter is that you might,

Understanding the Mind's Reaction to Violence

WHEN I WAS ATTACKED, I WAS SO DUMBFOUNDED THAT THE MAN WHO I thought loved me could hurt me like this that I couldn't begin to think how to react. I had no previous experience with violence and no experience defending myself. It took me a few minutes to figure out that he was not going to stop and that I was virtually helpless in defusing the situation. I have gone over and over these moments countless times, trying to figure out what I should have been thinking and doing while being attacked. First, I needed to know what was happening in my brain.

To learn more about the mind's reaction to fear, I began researching what happens in the brain when you face violence or the threat of violence. It was when I understood the basics of our cognitive response to fear—specifically, the mind's reaction to violence—that I realized cognitive training was a key element for all realistic training.

For many people who have faced violence, a common response is freezing or blacking out. Another common response is something along the lines of "My life flashed before my eyes." What this actually means is that because your mind can't come up with an immediate defense, it's searching through your memories, as if they were a giant database, for any kind of similar past experience that can provide a solution. It's looking for any kind of relevant event from your past that can tell it how to react. If you have never trained in self-defense with the correct instruction, your mind may come up blank, since you have no relevant experience to call upon. Without mental training, you really can't know how your mind will react in such a situation.

Personally, my mind was so overcome with trying to make sense of what was happening that I did freeze and was unable to come up with any viable self-defense response. But my experience doesn't have to be the norm. We can train our brains, through detailed visualization, to quickly break through the moment of freezing and indecision and to react. Freezing for a moment in a violent situation may indeed be inevitable, but you can train yourself to break through the "freeze phase" as quickly as possible.

and that your odds of survival and of escaping unharmed will go way up after you've read this book.

Every single concept, combative, and defense move in the following pages is included in the program I cover when working with a client, security agent, or celebrity in building the right foundation for self-defense. Throughout this book, I'll share self-defense details, tips, and strategies, but they will mean nothing if you aren't open to accepting the information from a perspective of reality. I know that you can take a class and mimic the instructor without really changing the way you think or truly absorbing the concepts. I see a lot of women who are able to do the moves in class and even perform them correctly under stress, but who still don't have the ability to use them on the street. What I want you to have is the perspective of reality, which simply means that you acknowledge your responsibility to learn these self-defense skills thoroughly enough to use if ever you're faced with a real, fear-inducing threat of violence. In reality, there won't be any time to step back and consider which motion would work best; you must be ready to act and react, effectively, in real time. And if that sounds daunting, don't worry—I will teach you how.

THE RACE REACTION MODEL

I designed the RACE (Recognize, Analyze, Compose, Execute) Reaction Model to help simplify many key findings, research, interviews with experts, and feedback from victims of violence, myself included. It has four phases, and, just as the name implies, you will learn how to race your reaction time when confronted with violence so that you can break through the freeze phase quickly and in time to defend yourself.

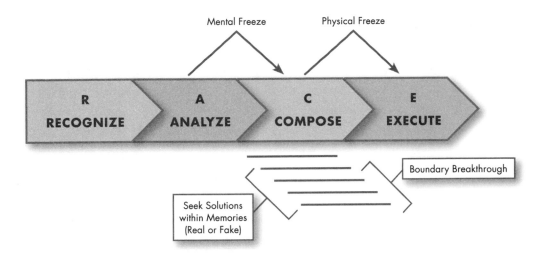

Phase 1: Recognize

Your mind first has to recognize the threat or attack in order to react to it. The ability to detect a threat comes from a trained level of situational awareness, which is simply being more aware of your surroundings. Your goal in this phase is to hone your situational awareness so you can detect the threat earlier and react to it faster.

Now, there is a way to be paranoid, and there is a way to live safely without compromising your quality of life. But it is also important to accept that even if you are cautious and avoid dangerous places, you may still be targeted and taken by surprise, as I was.

When you recognize a threat and adrenaline starts coursing through your body, your mind will try to help. Survival instinct takes over, and you will automatically transition into Phase 2.

Phase 2: Analyze

Whether or not you are tactically trained to do so, your mind will automatically analyze the threat. It will do its best to categorize the information it receives on the threat and work to identify the most important factors for survival. Your ability to do this effectively will depend on the work you put into following this training plan and preparing yourself through visualization and street drills.

Visualization training involves mentally putting yourself in a threatening situation and practicing identifying the factors that are most important for your survival. For example, when evaluating someone who may be a potential threat, an untrained person might concentrate on the aggressor's facial expression, but a tactically trained person will immediately look at his hands to see whether he is carrying a weapon, thus immediately determining a major factor in the threat. Another example: If facing the active attack of a man swinging a hook punch to one's face from a close distance, the untrained person would recognize a sudden movement and most likely attempt to see what is in the attacker's hands, while a trained person will focus on executing a strong and effective block before attempting to analyze what the attacker might be carrying in his hands. Later in this book, you'll do guided visualizations, and I'll prompt you to look for these kinds of factors.

The Analyze phase is the one that is most easily improved by mental training. With detailed visualization, you will be able to improve your natural reflexes so that your default physical reaction will temporarily stop or intercept an initial threat. But even if you move quickly through this phase, intercepting the initial threat is only the beginning of the battle. Your mind will then have to compose a defense, which brings us to Phase 3.

Phase 3: Compose

The composition phase involves your mind's computer calculating a plan of action. You may have heard of the phrase "fight or flight." As we learned above about the mind's reaction to violence, when victims describe their experience of freezing or having their life flash before their eyes, they are actually describing their mind's struggle to search for a solution. If you have been trained in self-defense and have visualized facing attacks, your mind will locate those memories, and you might pick "fight" and compose an action plan. If you haven't trained in self-defense and have no personal experience to draw upon, your mind may freeze from indecision and overwhelming fear.

Now, even if you know what to do and your mind composes a physical action, it doesn't necessarily mean that your body will move and react along with your mind. Have you ever experienced a total body freeze? By that I mean when your mind knows what to do and is telling your body to move, but your body feels stuck or like it's moving in slow motion. I have had this experience. That little voice in your head keeps on turning up the volume, but you don't react. So it is important to note that you will be faced with the challenge of overcoming the potential of both a mental freeze, where your mind doesn't know what to do, and a physical freeze, where your mind is responding but your body hasn't caught up yet. But don't worry—later in this book I'll give you solutions that will guide you to break through each potential freeze as fast as possible.

The good news is that you can activate this Compose phase to work for you, not against you. The solution is, again, visualization—creating fake "memories" of survival, so your mind practices the reactions you need to survive.

Visualizing being attacked and successfully implementing the moves you've learned will help your brain become adept at facing these attacks, both imagined and real. It is a very powerful training tool. Visualization of successful self-defense helps you know that your body has the ability to function, as required, to offer you protection. The power of visualization will also help you mold your body into a weapon of fitness—as you will begin to imagine yourself, in certain drills, striking a real attacker.

Phase 4: Execute

This is the phase in which you fight back. Once your mind recognizes the situation (Phase 1), analyzes the variables you need to react to (Phase 2), and composes your plan of survival (Phase 3), it is up to your body to carry through the operational plan (Phase 4). This is where all the work on the mat and in training sessions takes place, and this is why it's so important to train with good form.

The combatives, strikes, and stances you'll learn in the chapters ahead will come into play in the execution phase, turning your body into a weapon that you can rely on and training your muscles so that they retain the muscle memory necessary to work for your safety. I break down this formula further in "The Soteria Method Muscle Memory Training Guide," in Chapter 4.

HOW TO BUILD AN AUTHENTIC SURVIVAL MINDSET

When you have an authentic survival mindset, your mind is equipped with the tools necessary to formulate action plans against violent threats. As outlined in the RACE Reaction Model, a mind capable of executing self-defense techniques is one that can recognize a threat, analyze secondary factors, decide how to act, follow through with predetermined action, and continue to adapt to the threat by any means necessary.

In many ways, an authentic survival mindset is characterized as one that is not freaked out by the thought of violence but instead recognizes it for what it is: aggressive action from an individual who needs to be dealt with in a decisive manner. Those with a survival mindset don't contemplate the reasoning behind the threat (as I was stuck doing when my then-boyfriend attacked me without provocation) but will quickly and methodically determine the most effective plan of action—and execute it.

The good news is, it's simple to learn the skills that will give you an authentic survival mindset without making drastic negative changes to your sense of self. Having this survival mindset doesn't require you to live your life in paranoia or in a constant state of aggression. All it means is that you'll be prepared for anything, and you'll be taking responsibility for your own safety.

SURVIVAL MINDSET LIFE APPLICATION

Developing your own authentic survival mindset will, as it has for me, show you the stronger and more confident side of your personality, and its concepts can and will apply in various parts of your life to help you reach both personal goals and fitness goals. No matter what challenge you face or dream you want to achieve, the survival mindset will help you get there.

When you face violence, your survival mindset helps you to recognize and analyze the situation, then to compose an action plan and execute it until the threat no longer exists. And this same sequence of events will occur in your real life as well. Your survival mindset will allow you to face challenges and strive for your dreams with a clear action plan, using the same steps as in the RACE Reaction Model.

SURVIVAL MINDSET IN ACTION

You might be thinking to yourself, "I'd have no problem being aggressive if I was fighting to save my life." If so, great! But let's test that feeling. Try this simple exercise and pay attention to your first reaction when answering the question. So, let's say you are being attacked and you fear for the safety of your life. Assuming you knew how to perform an Eye Gouge (i.e., scooping an attacker's eyeball out of its socket), would you be able to eye-gouge your attacker to save your own life?

A This question is gross and I can't even think about it.
B No, because of physical, emotional, or spiritual boundaries.
C Maybe, if my life is threatened.
D Yes, definitely!

Okay, remember your answer. And now, I want you to answer the same question, but with a twist: you know the person attacking you.

A This question is gross and I can't even think about it.
B No, because of physical, emotional, or spiritual boundaries.
C Maybe, if my life is threatened.
D Yes, definitely!

Were your answers to both questions D, as they should be in the survival mindset? Or did your answer to the second question change? Your answer to the second question is the one that tells you the most about your current mindset and what mental boundaries may exist that could dictate or inhibit your ability to fight back in a life-threatening situation. If you know that you can protect yourself against someone you know and perhaps even love, then you have an authentic survival mindset.

Every person can discover mental boundaries in training; however, it is important to note that there can and usually will always be unknown boundaries you may have to face for the first time in a real-life threat or attack. These mental boundaries—whether it's a reluctance to inflict violence, a lack of belief in your own physical strength, or an idea that fighting back will only make it worse— might stop you from effectively fighting back.

Developing an authentic survival mindset will tackle those boundaries to eliminate any social, emotional, physical, and even spiritual blocks. Your ability to protect yourself is your right and your obligation. Ultimately, you are the only one who has control over your inhibitions, and you are the only one who can make the commitment to become your own security agent.

QUICK RECAP: A survival mindset is a frame of mind that operates with one objective, which is to survive at all costs. The first step to achieving this is taking a moment to accept that you could face violence for any reason, anywhere and at any time. Once you truly accept this, your mind will be hungry for a solution, and it starts with this book. Every minute you spend learning the concepts and practicing the moves in this book will help you absorb and integrate the tactics required to recognize and react to potentially violent situations. I am offering you a real plan to acquire self-defense skills that could save your life, but it is my responsibility to ensure that you are ready for what I am about to share with you.

COMMITMENT

And now, here's what I need from you. I can show you how to build a survival mindset and how to defend yourself no matter what life throws your way—but I will need your authentic commitment. Positive change happens only when you consistently demand it. So I need you to promise yourself right now that you will make this happen on a physical and mental level. It is important to understand that this method works with you and not for you. You can expect to gain only what you give.

What does that mean? All you have to do is follow, *really* follow, the plan that I have designed for you. I have already gone through the years of breaking bones, wrestling with sweaty opponents on the mat, and using my own body to run fitness experiments, time and again, to develop this method. All I am asking from you is to keep your word to follow through with it—no matter what. And you won't be doing it alone: I will help you every step of the way to focus your intent and determination.

Why am I pushing you to make this promise now? I need your commitment up front to make the most of this transformation because I have carefully designed a six-week program that will transform you into your own weapon of self-defense and fitness. This program is designed to fit within your lifestyle and enhance it in a positive way, but over the next six weeks you will face temptations, detours, and outside forces trying to push you off track. The only weapon that will save you is your promise to yourself—and to me—that you will continue.

I want you to take a moment to visualize yourself one year from now, three years, five years. Is there a particular lifestyle you want to achieve? How do you envision your life changing for the better? Do you want to be in better shape? Do you want to be a better protector of your children? Do you simply want to have the confidence to speak up more in meetings?

For my client Lucy, the motivator was motherhood. Lucy came to me soon after she got pregnant, saying that she wanted to get into shape so she wouldn't gain too much weight during pregnancy. I asked her to visualize her dream for her future, and she saw herself as a mother who was strong, fit, and independent enough to raise and protect her baby from anything she might face. Once she had identified this deep desire, she became much more focused on her workouts and developing her self-defense skills, motivated as she was by something so much more serious than just getting in shape. I'm happy to report that Lucy, now the proud mother of a one-year-old girl, is very adept at using improvised weapons and still trains with me twice a week. Should she ever be confronted by someone trying to snatch her daughter from her stroller, that would-be abductor will face a strong defense.

Take as long as you need to find the experience, feeling, or visual symbol that can formulate your commitment to changing your internal status quo. Also note that your motivation may evolve throughout the course of the transformation, but as long as you are in this for the right reason (for you), we can move forward and build your momentum for change.

Have you identified your own personal weapon of motivation and purpose? The answer should be yes before you move on. This driving force will help you get through some of the more challenging moments in the weeks ahead. Finding this motivating desire is key in developing your survival mindset.

AND NOW . . .

This journey of self-defense, fitness, and personal discovery will teach you to take control of your life and give you the power to fulfill your dreams. Your body will become a weapon—one that functions automatically and consistently. This workout could quite literally save your life. Are you ready? Let's begin.

HOW IT WORKS

▼

You are your own first and last line of defense. Now that you have accepted the possibility of facing violence for any reason, anywhere, and at any moment, it is time to implement a proactive solution for your safety. There happens to be a way that you can achieve this while also getting into the best shape of your life. This is where it all starts.

In the chapters to come, you'll begin a transformational journey. My signature fitness plan is designed to teach you to effectively strike an attacker—as well as to burn fat, build lean muscle, and sculpt the body for a powerful but feminine figure. *Weapons of Fitness* covers the same introductory combatives training program that I teach all my clients.

This book will transform you through strengthening, cardio, and nutrition. You'll get familiar with them and learn to love them! Your mission? To transform yourself into your own ultimate warrior goddess of safety. Together we are going to master three fields:

1 *Self-Defense:* Learn proper and effective striking combatives for self-defense concepts and applications that could save your life.

2 *Fitness:* Learn how to target and strengthen your body through fitness routines inspired by self-defense while developing the correct muscle memory for self-defense.

3 *Self-Discovery:* Adopt a Soteria Method–empowered lifestyle that will lead you to live a life that you love.

MOLDING YOUR WEAPONS

You are your own best weapon for a physical transformation. I'll show you how to mold your arms and legs into combative weapons powerful enough to save your life. I'll explain the technical foundation for building muscle memory as you practice and complete the movements throughout the workouts, and I'll tell you why form matters. Never underestimate the power of muscle memory. If you've been practicing correctly and you find yourself being attacked, your mind can compose the correct reaction and your body can execute it, with instinct and muscle memory taking over, and you can successfully defend yourself. But if you've been practicing with inconsistent and poor technique—limp hands instead of bladed, or a poor stance, or whatever—then even if your mind composes the correct reaction, your execution will most likely fail. From a self-defense perspective, the absolute worst thing you can do in practice is to strike wrong—and to repeatedly practice striking incorrectly. Practice everything perfectly!

COMBATIVES WILL BE USED in every phase of this workout. Why? I figure that since you are already spending the time exercising, you might as well maximize that time by learning self-defense too. And get psyched: You will see your body and feel your mindset transform as you work your way through the exercises. When I do these workouts, instead of focusing on how many reps I have left, as I would if I were just lifting weights or running laps, I am so focused on hitting the visualized targets that the workout is over before I know it.

THE CONCEPTS

I designed my workouts with five major concepts in mind:

1 *Define your goal.*
Take the time to really determine why you want to do these workouts and what you're hoping to achieve on this journey. Is your goal to learn to effectively strike someone and never miss a target? Is your goal to redefine health and happiness so that you can enjoy life? Is your goal to finally burn fat and sculpt your ultimate feminine figure? These are just some questions to get you thinking, but once you've identified that underlying goal and begun to build your survival mindset, you'll be unshakable.

2 *Be consistent.*
Make sure you're doing each combative with absolutely perfect form. For every position and physical movement, first use a full-length mirror as your training partner to gain an awareness of your movements and to work toward consistency.

3 *Boost muscle memory.*
Once you are sure that you can accurately hit the same place every time, with a consistent reach and without the help of a mirror, transition away from the mirror and begin to feel the correct technical execution of your movements.

4 *Try it for real.*
After you have practiced a move enough without a mirror to know that your combatives are accurate and powerful, it's time to find a training partner for the real-world application of these moves. Having real-world experience in defending yourself from a perceived threat is crucial to helping you move through the Compose phase of an attack. I will take you through great drills that you can do at home alone or with a training partner.

5 *Visualize.*
Real practice of these moves with a training partner is excellent, but whether or not you have a training partner, I want you to visualize the moves as well. By closing your eyes and focusing your mind on facing a realistic, threatening situation and nullifying it with your actions, you'll force yourself to pay

attention to details. Visualization will condition your mind to create the "fake experiences" that you want to insert into your memory, so that when your life flashes before your eyes and your brain seeks relevant experiences to draw from, your mind will find these visualized experiences and know what to do. (Please note that a visualization guide will be provided later on in this book.)

WEAPONS OF FITNESS BREAKDOWN

Here's how this book is going to work. First, I'm going to walk you through all the combatives that will be used in the workouts. I want you to practice them in slow motion, in front of a mirror, until you know what you're doing and are ready to bring them up to normal speed.

I'll break down exactly how three major weapons of fitness—strengthening, cardio, and nutrition—will play equally crucial roles in your physical transformation. Then you'll take a short fitness placement test, based on six classic exercises you're probably familiar with: the squat, the lunge, the push-up, the sit-up, the plank, and the burpee. Your performance on the fitness placement test will determine your starting point: beginner, intermediate, advanced, or for you wild women out there, advanced plus.

And at last it's time for the main event! You'll move on to the workouts, where you'll do the combatives quickly and in fast sequences, as you would if you were being attacked (and this will give you a great cardio workout too). Promise me six weeks of faithfully following my workouts and sticking to my nutrition plans, and I promise you transformation. Every two weeks, I will provide you with a new cardio combative challenge, a new toning routine, and some new nutrition tips and secrets that have allowed me to feel strong, empowered, and ready to attack the life that I want. Why two-week progressions? I want you to have the time to properly develop the combatives so that they become second nature. You know how important muscle memory is; don't skimp on it.

I'm Right There with You

YOU'RE NOT GOING THROUGH THIS ALONE. THROUGHOUT THE BOOK, I HIGH-light how I overcame some of my personal challenges. Ultimately, I want to help you protect those dreams and ambitions we identified in Chapter 2 and to show you that this workout has many valuable aspects beyond those of safety, fitness, and health.

CREATING, LIVING, AND LOVING YOUR LIFE THROUGH SELF-DEFENSE

Studying self-defense saved me when I was in a dark place, but redefining self-defense for myself is what helped me learn to love life again. Remember our new definition of "self-defense": training to attack the life you want, not letting life attack you. And to protect your ideal life, you first have to create it. Chapter 13 outlines my personal secrets for having the ability to wake up, knock out my fears, and attack life.

ONE FINAL THING before we begin: thank you. Thank you for standing up for yourself, and thank you for wanting to learn how to defend your life, with your own inner Soteria goddess. And now get ready, because you are in for a fun fight for life!

MOLDING YOUR WEAPON

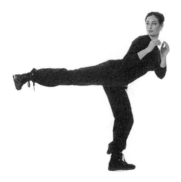

STANCES

▼

I t's time to get physical, and it's time to get tactical. In these next few pages, I'll show you my favorite stances and how to apply my muscle memory training guide so that you will have perfect form every time. I'll also share some strategic secrets that have allowed me to overcome the physical and mental freezes associated with fear and a surge of adrenaline. The concepts I'll arm you with will make you reactive to the unknown and will give you the ability to adapt to the always-changing dynamics of personal defense. Simplicity means survival when it comes to self-defense—and I'll now show you just how simple striking someone can be.

THE POSITIVE ANGLE APPROACH

First, let's talk about angles. And no, I don't mean physical angles. When I say "positive angle," I'm talking about the advantage or positive opportunity the attacker and the situation present to your defense. Training to recognize your positive advantage in every situation conditions your mind to flip into a proactive and tactical survival mindset, instead of one of fear and victimization.

How did this come about? I realized in training that no matter what attack or situation I was facing, I had to uncover the positive angle—and there always is one. What does this actually mean, in practice? Many perceived self-defense disadvantages, especially for women, are actually gifts, provided you train to make them work for you.

For example, as a woman, when you face a male attacker, he is likely to be bigger and more muscular than you are. So you're likely already operating within the underdog frame of mind. This forces you to rely on mechanics, leverage, and your self-defense training—as opposed to the attacker, who will likely be overconfident in his physical superiority alone and won't be expecting you to be able to outsmart his attack.

Let's look at another situation. Say an attacker makes physical contact with your body. This may be scary, but it's also your positive angle; every time your attacker makes contact with you and grabs you, he forces himself into a fixed position, which gives you the opportunity to work from a reference position. And another benefit: If he's holding you with one arm, he's given up that arm as a striking weapon! So the positive here is that he has brought you to a range or distance in which you have options to control and strike, while he's actually limiting his options by using one hand to hold you.

From a self-defense perspective, I will uncover the positive angles in all the defenses and situations in this book. When you finish this book, you'll realize that every challenge, no matter how daunting, gives you a positive angle—and exploring those can lead you to new possibilities in life.

BREAKING DOWN AND BUILDING UP

Whether you are a competitive boxer, you used to fight with your siblings, or you have never thrown a punch in your life, you'll almost certainly have to unlearn form and style from previous training or assumptions. Many of my students express frustration at this point, but don't worry or give up. My combative training guide is a concept-based design that has proven to be effective, retainable, and easily ingrained into your muscle memory. Kicking bad habits is a small price to pay.

THE SOTERIA METHOD MUSCLE MEMORY TRAINING GUIDE

As you go through the stances in this chapter and continue to learn combatives throughout this book, use this muscle memory training guide for each and every one of them. That way, if you ever need to execute these moves, at least you won't have to think about them first.

1 *Understand the Why:* First understand the objective of the position, strike, or tactic and why it could help save your life. Imagine a few scenarios in which you would apply the combative or tactic. This will wake up your survival mindset so that it can take in the information to use as a realistic application.

2 *Know the What:* Find out what positions and movements work for your body to achieve the self-defense concept, tactic, or objective. For example, in the chapters to come, I will break down how to learn combatives using three simple factors that will ensure a consistent technical execution and accuracy against all targets.

3 *Visual Referencing:* Perform the required movements or position in front of a mirror to gain visual consistency. Gradually increase your speed by intervals of 10 to 20 percent once you've achieved correct form and technique. Remember, your technique will be compromised when you are performing under the adrenaline state in a real-life situation, so the higher the level of technical consistency you can maintain, the better your technique will be on the street.

4 *Blind Referencing:* Step away from the mirror or close your eyes in between practice drills to begin feeling what the proper form feels like. Gradually increase your speed by intervals of 10 to 20 percent once you've achieved correct form and technique.

5 *Physical Application:* Apply the tactics in drills and with a training partner if possible.

6 Visualization: Close your eyes and visualize yourself performing the tactics in real locations from your daily life. Experience applying the defense in the best-case and the worst-case scenarios to fill your survival mindset memory box.

Let's get going!

STANCES

First, you'll need to master these three self-defense training stances: my classic Survival Stance, Hidden Survival Stance, and Off-Guard Stance. Each stance has a different objective and purpose as it relates to self-defense strategy and training, and you'll be practicing your combatives from these stances in the next chapter. So whether you're building your base of balance or conditioning your mind and body to react from the vulnerable position of being caught off-guard, these stances are crucial, because you need to be able to maintain your balance and shift your weight in the blink of an eye. Practice the stances until you can step into them easily and quickly.

✸ Survival Stance

Objective • To maintain your balance while physically defending yourself.

Description • I consider the Survival Stance to be my fail-safe position when I'm defending myself. The angled position of the feet with the bladed upper body and shield-like arm position makes it the best base to work from when applying protective tactics. "Blading your body" refers to facing your attacker on a diagonal so that you become a smaller target, as one side of your body is aligned behind the other side.

Timing • You don't want to get into Survival Stance too early. Until the attacker has actively engaged in his attack or until you confirm the need to act proactively in your defense, you don't want him to know that you are preparing to escape or fight back, as that will send a strong body language message of your prior training

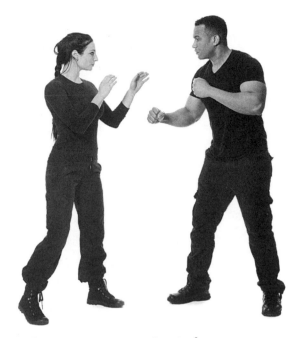

or, at the very least, your will to fight back. If your attacker can tell that you are going to fight back, he might increase the level of violence or prepare a backup plan. Either way, you want to work with the element of surprise and aim to catch the attacker off guard—a key principle in the Soteria Method. When you do decide to become active, your home base position should be this stance.

Follow these simple steps to find your own Survival Stance. Try both sides to determine which is your dominant side. Work through your dominant side first to understand the concepts and combatives before training your other side.

Below are the simple steps that will lead you to discover your own Survival Stance. Reference the images below to help you successfully achieve every step.

Finding Your Personal Survival Stance

Step 1: Put both feet together.

Step 2: Turn both feet 45 degrees to the right to successfully blade your body.
Blading your body refers to your turning the front of your body on the diagonal so that you are a smaller target in front of your threat.

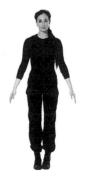
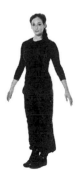
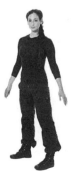
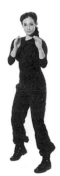
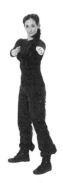

Step 1   Step 2   Step 3   Step 4   Step 5

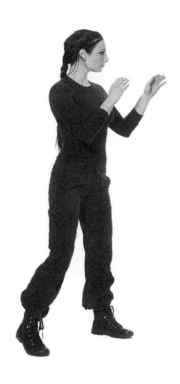

Step 3: Take one step on that diagonal so that your feet are slightly wider than shoulder-width apart.

Step 4: Raise your arms to shoulder level and maintain your bladed body so that your rear leg pulls that same shoulder back.

Step 5: Relax the elbows, keep them in front of your body, and keep your hands open. Make sure to keep your hands up to guard your face.

TIPS

Balance Your Weight: You want your weight to be centered. Test this by lifting the heel of your rear foot off the ground and making sure that you don't transition your weight onto your front leg. My students learn how to maintain the Survival Stance by imagining a red laser beam constantly shooting down from their spine, even when they transition between feet.

Protect Your Face: Keeping your arms placed at shoulder level provides a central location to react from and also allows your hands to shield your face and body. If you find you are dropping your hands, keep your fingertips touching your cheekbones until you naturally hold your hands up in front of you.

Keep Your Hands Open: The Survival Stance requires your hands to be open because you never know what type of attack you will face. For example, you might have to block a punch or grab the barrel of the gun. If your hands are curled into fists, you'll lose precious milliseconds uncurling them.

Blade Your Body: By blading the body (having one side behind the other), you make yourself a smaller target and also cover and protect more of your body.

SURVIVAL STANCE DRILLS

Muscle Memory Drill

Stand in front of the mirror and get into Survival Stance. Take note of the visual references such as the distance between your feet, your bladed upper body, where your elbows line up, and the level of your fingertips in relation to your cheekbones. Return to regular standing position. Then move back into Survival Stance and make sure your form is perfect. Practice this until you get into this stance consistently on both sides. Then do it with your eyes closed, and when you open your eyes, check to see that the position is correct.

Subway Drill

If you take the subway or bus, I recommend testing your stance by letting go of the handrails and maintaining your balance in your Survival Stance as the car moves between stations or stops. Your feet will adjust to maintain your balance. If you don't use the subway or bus, you can ask a friend to lightly attempt to push you off balance from all directions as you try to hold your stance.

✳ Hidden Survival Stance

Objective • To obtain a safety stance while confirming a threat.

Description • The Survival Stance sends a strong message to the attacker that you are willing to fight back, which gives away your element of surprise. If you suspect or have already confirmed a threat but don't yet want your would-be attacker to know that you've been trained in self-defense, then you want to immediately get into your Hidden Survival Stance.

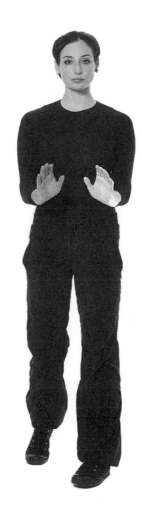

Timing • I want you to train for this stance to be your fail-safe response the second you recognize a threat. Your Hidden Survival Stance won't be perceived as a stance of survival. Instead, it will portray a submissive and frightened body language but will actually allow you to get centered and ready for a possible attack, even as you keep your attacker's guard down and leverage this element of surprise when you do take action.

Overcoming the Freeze • In addition to learning the physical default stance, I want you to train saying the word "okay" as you transition into this stance. This simultaneous reaction of the mind and body will better help you overcome any initial physical and or mental freeze. The word "okay" will also make your attacker think that you are submissive and cooperative, meaning he'll let his guard down even further.

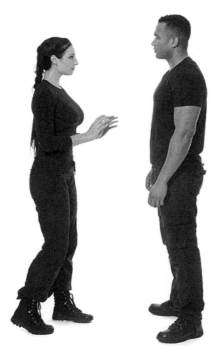

Hidden Survival Stance

Hidden Survival Stance How-To

As you can see in the photo opposite, I am covertly doing my Hidden Survival Stance. Here's how to get into your Hidden Survival Stance:

Step 1: Bring your rear leg slightly back.

Step 2: Bring your hands up to your sternum, but in a pleading and calming manner.

Step 3: Mentally prepare to fight (which your attacker will never see).

Specific Drill • Stand in front of the mirror and pretend to hide your full Survival Stance from yourself, which will help lead you to your personal Hidden Survival Stance.

✳ Off-Guard Stance

Objective • To condition the cognitive recognition and physical self-defense reaction from the state of being unaware or caught off guard.

Description • No matter how prepared you are, there will always be moments when you have let someone enter into your personal space and something goes wrong. Whether it's a partner, a coworker, a friend, or an acquaintance, sometimes people get too close, and before you realize it, you find yourself vulnerable. For this reason, you will be practicing combatives from a totally neutral stance, as though you've been caught completely off guard.

Timing • You will use this stance to fight only when you've been caught completely by surprise.

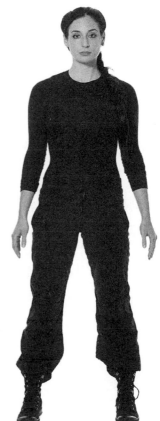

Off-Guard Stance

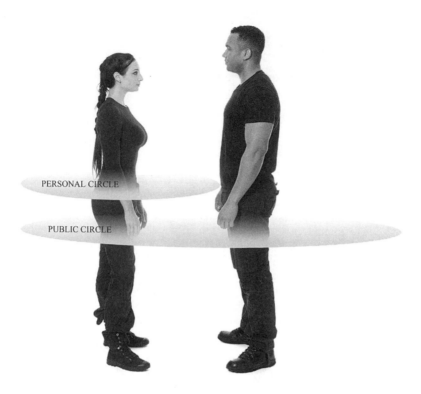

PERSONAL CIRCLE

PUBLIC CIRCLE

In the diagram above, I have outlined two personal circles of safety. Your "personal circle of safety" is a comfortable distance between you and a person you are holding a conversation with. I recommend keeping your personal circle of safety at a striking distance—by which I mean that if you were to fully execute a strike using your arm, you could make contact easily. The second, outer circle is your "public circle." This is a comfortable range between you and someone you don't know. I like to make sure I can at least kick someone when maintaining this public circle of safety. However, there will be situations, as in the subway or other crowded areas, in which you'll have no choice about people invading your safety circles—hence the need to train from an Off-Guard Stance.

Specific Drill • Visualize at least ten scenarios of people respecting and then invading your personal circle of safety to clearly define these tactical boundaries for yourself mentally. That way, when people do invade it in real life, your hackles will rise instantly.

✳ Traveling in Survival Stance

Objective • To maintain your Survival Stance and essentially your balance as you transition and cover distance.

Description • You want to have the ability to adjust your range or distance, simultaneously travel and strike, and ultimately stay on your feet against a variety of pressures.

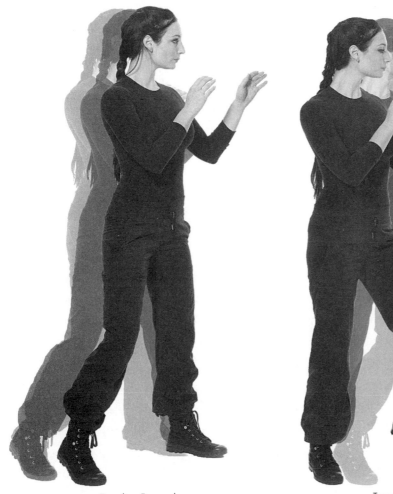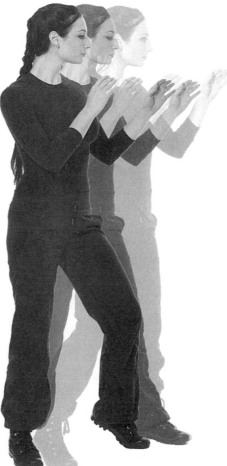

Traveling Forward   Traveling Backward

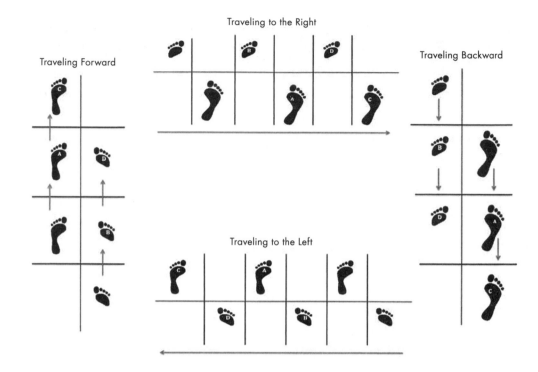

Traveling Forward

Traveling to the Right

Traveling Backward

Traveling to the Left

Traveling in Survival Stance How-To • To maintain the Survival Stance while traveling, you must cover approximately the same amount of distance with both feet; otherwise, you will gallop at high speed and risk tripping and falling.

Specific Drill • Travel in all directions. Travel forward, backward to the left, and to the right. Make sure that the foot of the leg that is closest to the direction you are traveling remains flat and that the far-side leg has the heel raised. For example, if you're moving forward and your left leg is forward, your left foot should be flat on the ground with each step, and your right foot's heel should be raised.

✳ Breaking the Angle

Objective • To remove yourself from the direct line of the threat.

Description • One of the best defenses against an attack is to not be there when it hits. Breaking your angle at the right time will literally remove your body from the path of the attacker. Learning how to break the angle will also help you stay facing the attacker and preventing him from getting behind you, another big concept in the Soteria Method, which is that you never want to expose your back to an attacker, even for a split second.

Timing • Break the angle whenever your attacker moves. When he moves, you move.

Breaking the Angle How-To • To break the angle, pivot on the ball of your front foot and rotate your body 90 degrees, moving your back foot.

Specific Drill • Attempt to break the angle by 90 degrees. If you are in a room, use each wall as a new angle. Practice breaking the angle to the right and to the left.

Partner Drill • Face a partner. One partner will be the aggressor and change direction while the other partner will attempt to maintain the distance between the two and not let the other get to the rear side. If you don't have a partner, it is almost as effective to visualize someone there.

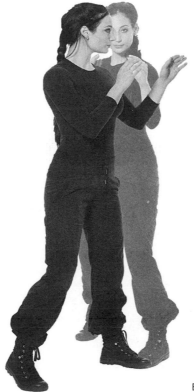

Breaking the Angle to the Left

UPPER-BODY COMBATIVES

▼

Now you know that the moment you realize that you're going to have to defend yourself, you need to get into your Hidden Survival Stance or Survival Stance. No matter whether you're closing in, blocking a knife attack, or fighting to stay up on your feet, your Survival Stance is your home base. Make sure these positions feel natural and easy.

Now that you've mastered the stances, we're going to turn our focus to combatives. Get ready to become your own weapon of personal protection.

COMBATIVE THEORY

As I noted, a combative is a strike, and a strike is you driving a surface area of your body through the vulnerable target on the attacker—when it is available. What do I mean by "through" the target? The same thing your elementary school softball coach meant when he told you to run "through" first base after you hit the ball.

The more velocity you have when you make the strike, the more powerful and effective it will be.

I have taught thousands of women how to effectively use upper-body and lower-body combative strikes against attackers by equipping them to adapt to the unpredictable realities on the street. Being armed with both the right idea and the right moves immediately and significantly increases your chances of surviving a variety of attacks. And no matter how unprepared you feel to strike someone, you can train and build correct muscle memory based on a consistent range of motion that will ensure that you always make contact with your intended target.

What's the objective of a combative? To disrupt the attacker's thought process. That's it. You are not aiming to inflict pain or to knock him out; neither of these results can be guaranteed. For example, say that you kick your attacker in the groin with the goal of inflicting pain. You might expect him to collapse to the ground and yell in pain, and he very well might. However, your attacker could be on drugs or have a high tolerance level for pain (or even an inability to feel pain). If you target his groin, you need to be prepared to keep fighting if he doesn't collapse.

Most male attackers, however, will at the very least flinch when you strike them in the groin, and take an extra millisecond or two to react, buying you some time to follow up with more combatives or to run away. An added bonus: If you've kicked him in the groin and he has bent over even a little bit, you have also shortened his original frame of height, which now grants you, as a (probably) smaller defender, access to the level of his face.

What's important here is that you strategically train for outcomes that you can more likely guarantee and that will always have an added bonus for you. If you focus on successfully disrupting the thought process, then you can adapt in the time that it takes him to recover. Coming from this perspective will simplify your actions and place you in the driver's seat, not the backseat. Please pay attention to this and retain this concept, because I am not going to show you a fancy combination of combatives and leave you hoping for the best. Instead, I will show you how to ensure that your combatives make contact with the targets and that your mental effort is in the "adaptive mindset," where you are already anticipating the next move to neutralize the life-threatening situation.

3-FACTOR COMBATIVE THEORY

To help you remember the crucial basics, I have simplified striking into what I call the 3-Factor Combative Theory.

Factor One: Target

What target is available and most vulnerable? Ultimately, the primary target on the upper half of the attacker is the eyes or face. The primary lower target is his groin.

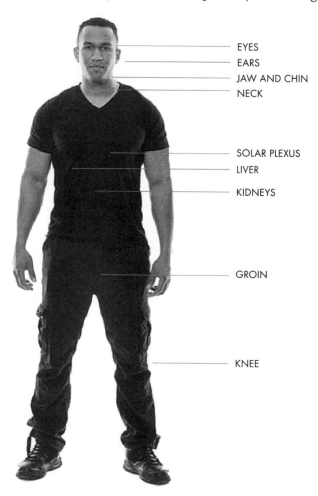

EYES
EARS
JAW AND CHIN
NECK

SOLAR PLEXUS
LIVER
KIDNEYS

GROIN

KNEE

By "primary" target, I mean one with a high probability of access or availability and a high level of effectiveness in disrupting an attacker's thoughts. The image opposite outlines the most vulnerable targets on a male attacker. Note that although most attacks against women are committed by men, a female attacker is still a possibility; however, the tactics I am outlining will remain the same, regardless of an attacker's gender.

Factor Two: Surface Area

Which surface area will you use to strike with? In general, you want to use an area that is strong and tough, such as the heel of the palm, as opposed to the knuckles of the fist. The elbow is another great choice, as the bone is much stronger there than elsewhere on the arm. But again, which surface you use will be dependent on the situation and what you can reach your attacker with, not what you like or think is the best sequence to remember. Some of the strongest surfaces include the heel of the palm, the elbow, the knee, and the heel of the foot. See the next page for an illustration of surface area options.

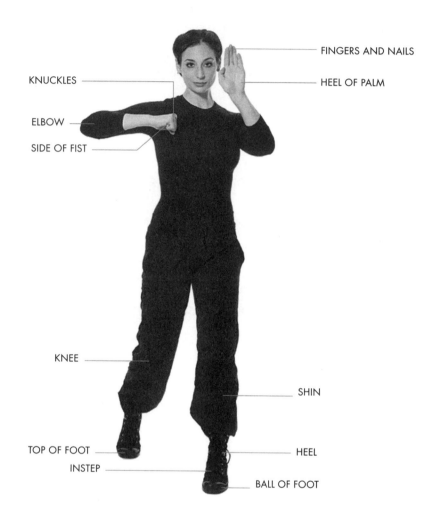

FINGERS AND NAILS

KNUCKLES

HEEL OF PALM

ELBOW

SIDE OF FIST

KNEE

SHIN

TOP OF FOOT

HEEL

INSTEP

BALL OF FOOT

Factor Three: Range of Motion

I want to highlight two primary movements that allow you to reach your optimal and full range of motion and obtain consistency and power in your technique: the direct upper-body power source called the Combative Twist, which I'll discuss later in this chapter, lets you generate as much power as possible by placing the force of your entire body behind each strike; and the lower-body power source called the Hip Thrust, which I'll cover in the next chapter.

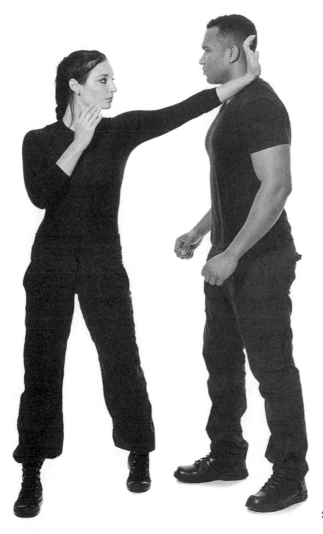

Striking through the Target

COMBATIVE RANGE

Combative range is the space between you and your attacker in which you can make physical contact with using a combative. This is why muscle memory is crucial. The attacker's profile will change—his height, physical reach, pain tolerance, athletic ability, and natural reflexes—but the one thing that won't change is the way you execute your combatives.

Each person has a unique range of motion, and learning how to strike consistently will help you build an awareness of and a sixth sense for effective striking distances. Based on this muscle memory, you will able to focus on the strategic and tactical execution of your combatives to adapt to changing situations—rather than focusing on the technical execution of combatives themselves. As we cover each combative, I will give the general range, but ultimately you will realize at what distance each combative best works for you. Here are the four types of ranges:

Long Range

This is the range when your attacker is far enough away that you can't reach him with your arms but with your legs. The combatives you'll employ at this range include those with your longest reach, such as the Push Kick, Side Kick, Snap Kick, and Rear Kick.

Medium Range

This range, when the attacker is within arm's reach, is the most effective distance at which to use the upper-body combatives that require a full extension of the arms, such as Straight Strikes (Closed Fist, Palm Strikes), Eye Gouging, and Raking.

Control Range

You'll know when you are in the control range, because you will be able to easily grab your attacker's face. It is the closest range of distance that can exist between a defender and an attacker while standing—and this is the range you actually *want* to get to if you have no option but to close in and neutralize the attack. Combatives for this range include Defensive Elbows, Defensive Knees, Shin Kicks, Eye Gouging, Control Holds, Disarms, and more.

Ground Range

This means you're on the ground. You want to avoid this range at all costs, but at the same time, as a woman, you have to accept that the ground range is probably where your attacker wants you. Thankfully, at this range you can still apply all the concepts and tactics from this book, and even modified versions of all your combatives. Applications to ground survival and rape prevention include Ground Push Kicks, Side Kicks, Eye Gouging, and Defensive Elbows (all angles).

As we transition into the core combatives of the workout, remember to apply the concepts from "The Soteria Method Muscle Memory Training Guide," in Chapter 4, to each combative in addition to the specific drills I recommend.

✸ Combative Twist: Your Upper-Body Power Source

Objective • The power comes from the torso and the core of the body. The twisting motion of the torso lets you put your full body weight behind your strikes and allows you to generate much greater power. The striking arm also has an impact, so look at the arm itself as the weapon, and look at the twist as your pulling the trigger to generate force.

Combative Twist How-To • Starting in Survival Stance, pull your near-side shoulder and hip (the shoulder and hip closest to your attacker) forward sharply so that your body rotates powerfully. Make sure to align your shoulders with your hipbones so that your body rotates as a unit, and to keep your ankle and knee pointed in the same direction. This will force you to pivot on the ball of your front foot. Welcome to your full range of motion from your near side—that closest to your attacker.

Now let's find our full range of motion from our rear side. Starting in Survival Stance, lead your rotation from your rear shoulder. Keeping the hip and knee in line, drive your rear shoulder and hip forward powerfully, pivoting on the ball of

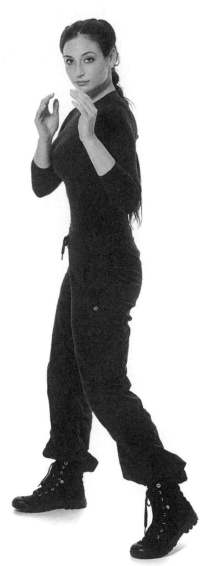

Near-Side Combative Twist

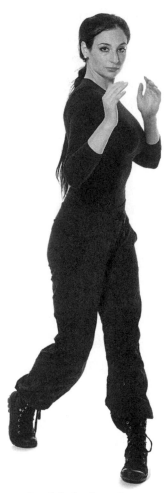

Rear-Side Combative Twist

the rear foot. Common mistakes that I see with my students are that they will lean in or transition their weight onto the leg that is not twisting. When doing combatives, make sure to keep your weight centered equally between both feet.

***Weapons of Fitness* Benefit** • Practicing twisting your body to generate power will tighten and strengthen your core to help you get that flat stomach you've always wanted. And when you increase the speed of your strikes—as you will in both the cardio combative challenges and the burnout intervals (high-speed, repetitive combative rounds that we will be integrating into our *Weapons of Fitness* workouts)—you'll start to see some serious strengthening. This quick twist forces your abdominals and obliques to help rotate your shoulders, so you can extend your arms and generate the greatest amount of force.

STRAIGHT STRIKE COMBATIVES

A straight strike is a combative that operates within in your sagittal plane of motion. It is the fastest path and the least telegraphic. In other words, you are leveraging off of speed as you execute strikes that travel on a direct path, as opposed to striking on a circular path, which takes more time and runs the risk of telegraphing (or prematurely showing your attacker) your intent.

✳ Palm Strike

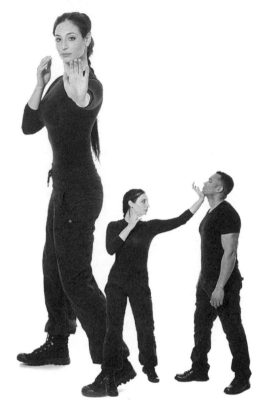

Near-Side Palm Strike

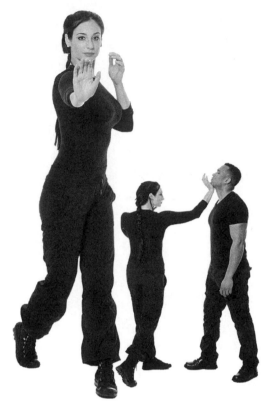

Rear-Side Palm Strike

Target • Face, chin, nose, eyes

Surface Area • The heel of your palm

Range of Motion • Combative Twist

Combative Range • Medium

Palm Strike How-To • Drive the heel of your palm through a point on your attacker's face, with a full Combative Twist to generate power.

***Weapons of Fitness* Benefit** • Core and upper body when performing burn-outs or speed drills

Variation • Circle Path—if you have limited wrist mobility or find yourself close to your attacker, you can circle the heel of your palm to his nose, chin, or face. In other words, you can still prepare the heel of your palm as the surface area, but for this variation, by adding a slight bend in the elbow joint, you enable a circular path to make contact with the target. The Combative Twist still applies to generate force.

How to Make a Fist

MANY VARIATIONS OF STRAIGHT STRIKES INVOLVE USING THE FIST, THE WEB OF your hand, or the fingertips. For myself, I have trained the heel of my palm to be my default or primary surface area, as it is stronger and less fragile for self-defense. In this next section, I highlight alternate combatives that use different surface areas so you will have extra "weapons" to call upon. First, I'll break down how to make a fist, shown in the images below. As you can see, you want to curl the fingers so that you have a nice flat surface, and then wrap your thumb around your fist to close the grip.

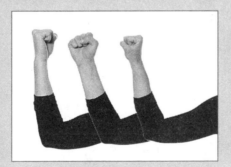

✹ Fist Strike

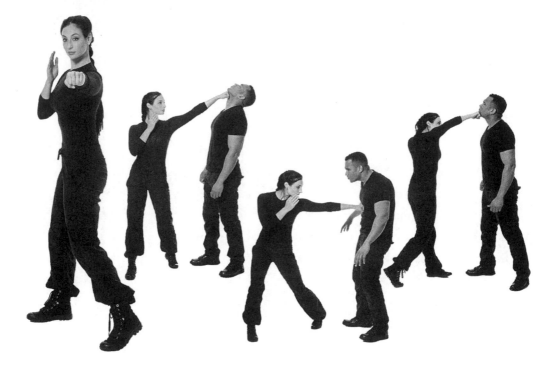

Target • Face, chin, nose, solar plexus, groin

Surface Area • Knuckles of fist

Range of Motion • Combative Twist

Combative Range • Medium

Fist Strike How-To • Drive the knuckles of your fist through the attacker's body using a full Combative Twist to generate power.

***Weapons of Fitness* Benefit** • Core and upper body when doing burnouts or speed drills

Comments • Whatever your height, do not consider it a barrier to hitting targets at different levels. Whether you are five feet and can make direct contact with someone's groin or five foot ten and want to hit lower to target the solar plexus, you can do it. It's great to train doing Fist Strikes at different target levels to condition yourself to adjust to possible variations in a real-life situation.

✳ Web Strike

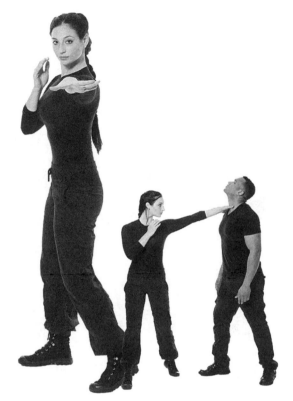

Near-Side Web Strike

Target · Throat

Surface Area · Web of hand

Range of Motion · Combative Twist

Combative Range · Medium/Control

Web Strike How-To · Drive the web of your hand through the attacker's neck using a full Combative Twist to generate power.

***Weapons of Fitness* Benefit** · Core and upper body when performing burn-outs or speed drills

Comments · This combative uses a higher level of force and is really effective when you are working from a Control Hold, in which you secure the arm of your attacker by trapping him close to your body (see pages 106–8 for more on Control

Holds), where you are in the control range or when you have a direct opening to the attacker's throat.

✷ Combative Flick

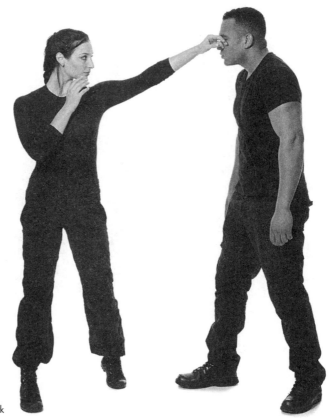

Near-Side Combative Flick

Target • Eyes

Surface Area • Fingertips

Range of Motion • Combative Twist

Combative Range • Medium

Combative Flick How-To • As you extend for a straight combative, relax your fingers, flicking your wrist while driving your hand forward. By aiming for the attacker's eyes, you can temporarily disrupt his vision and therefore his thought process—giving you time to launch into your next strategic move.

***Weapons of Fitness* Benefit** • Core and upper body when performing burnouts or speed drills

✴ Hammer Fist

Target • Face, temple, back of the head

Surface Area • Outer surface of fist

Range of Motion • The Hammer Fist is very practical because it can be executed from a wide range of angles. To clarify, the angle represents one of the many paths that the fist can take in order to hit open targets on the attacker's body. This includes Downward Hammer Fists, Angled Hammer Fists, and Backhand Hammer Fists. I have outlined below the angles that will be used in the workouts.

Combative Range • Medium/Control (depending on angle used)

Comments • This strike can be performed on multiple target levels, depending on the physical reaction of the attacker and how quickly he ends up on his knees or physically compromised. The Hammer Fist is a relatively safe way to use your fists to make contact with a target, as the surface area is strong and leaves you less vulnerable to any injuries. To warm up and find the best surface area for a Hammer Fist, bang the outside of your fist on a table or door. This type of movement will lead us into our first angle, which is a Downward Hammer Fist.

✺ Downward Hammer Fist

Target • Face in general, nose, jaw, back of head

Surface Area • Side of fist

Range of Motion • Combative Twist

Combative Range • Medium

Downward Hammer Fist How-To

1 Starting in Survival Stance, raise your near-side hand just above eye level. Curl your fingers to turn your hand into a fist.

2 Twist from your core as you drive the outside of your fist into the chin or nose of your attacker.

3 Strike through the target, continuing into his body as if you want to strike into his chest. Remember not to drop your other arm.

4 Immediately return to Survival Stance.

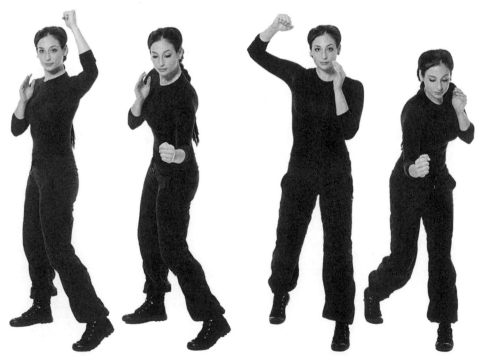

Near-Side Downward Hammer Fist   Rear-Side Downward Hammer Fist

✳ Angled Hammer Fist

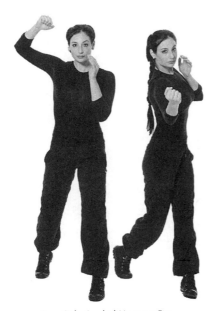

Rear-Side Angled Hammer Fist

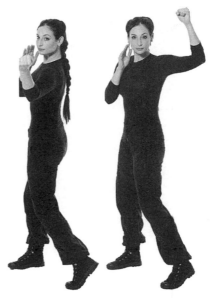

Near-Side Angled Hammer Fist

Target • Face in general, temple, jaw

Surface Area • Side of fist

Range of Motion • Combative Twist

Combative Range • Medium

Angled Hammer Fist How-To

1 Starting in Survival Stance, raise your near-side hand just above eye level, but this time, slightly open your arm to set up the diagonal angle.

2 Twist as your drive your surface area into the side of the head or jaw of your attacker.

3 Strike through the target, continuing into his body as if you want to hit the opposite side of his shoulder or chest.

4 Immediately return to Survival Stance.

✳ Back Hammer Fist

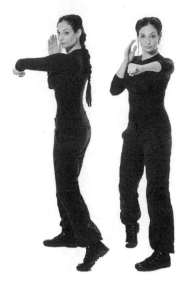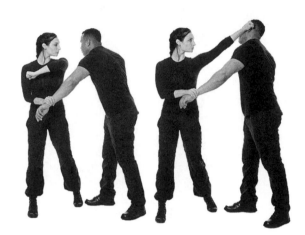

Target • Face in general, temple, jaw

Surface Area • Side of fist

Range of Motion • Combative Twist

Combative Range • Medium

Back Hammer Fist How-To

1 This variation has a slightly different starting position. Begin in the Off-Guard Stance perpendicular to the attacker. Once you've located the target, raise your near-side fist so that your forearm is parallel to the ground and your elbow is bent at a 90-degree angle.

2 Twist as you drive your surface area into the side of the head or jaw of your attacker.

3 To strike through the target, continue driving your fist past his head as if you are aiming for someone standing right beside him.

4 Immediately return to Survival Stance.

Comments • This is a great primary combative to practice. Many women use it as their go-to counter-combative because it gives them a combination of power and reach when facing a much larger attacker.

✳ Low Hammer Fist

Target • Groin

Surface Area • Side of fist

Range of Motion • Lateral Hip Shift

Combative Range • Control

Low Hammer Fist How-To

1 Simply shift your hips and simultaneously raise your fist.

2 Extend your fist downward to make contact with the attacker's groin.

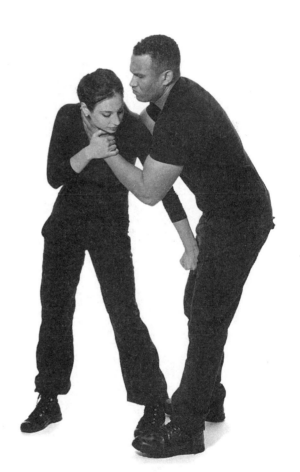

Comments • This is extremely effective to use when you are facing an attack from the rear, such as a bear hug or choke hold, in which the attacker's body is close to yours. In the image at right, I am applying a Low Hammer Fist against a side choke hold to help create distance against his close grip. Even though my arm is technically pinned, the positive angle in this situation is that I still have mobility in my hips, and by shifting my hips, I give my arm the space and opportunity to execute a Hammer Fist to the groin.

✻ Raking

Target • Eyes, face

Surface Area • Fingertips

Range of Motion • Combative Twist

Combative Range • Medium/Control

Raking How-To • The Raking execution is similar to that of the angle variations of the Hammer Fist, but with a different surface area. In this case, your surface area is your fingers; you're going to scratch your attacker's face with your nails, like a cat would in a catfight. When you do rake, make sure that you place ten-

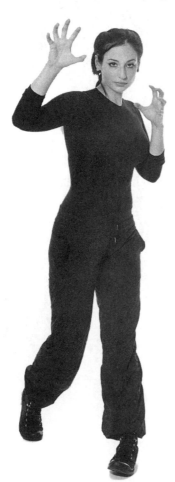

sion in your fingers. Your hand position should be open, as if you are holding an invisible ball.

Comments • This is a great combative to use when you are close enough to target the eyes. At the very least, this will disrupt your attacker's thought process and even temporarily compromise his sight.

✳ Eye Gouge

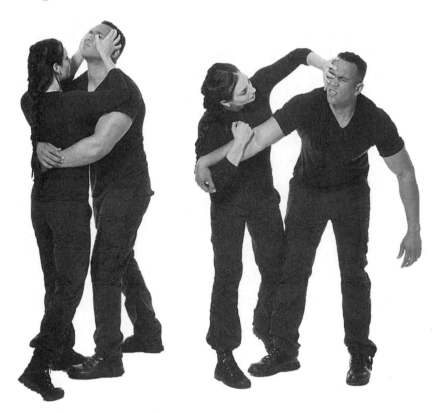

Target · Eyes

Surface Area · Fingertips

Range of Motion · Angled Arm Extension

Combative Range · Control

Eye Gouge How-To · If you're facing your attacker head-on and he's using both arms to hold you, then place both thumbs into his eye sockets to scoop out the eyeballs. In addition to completing the Eye Gouge, you can be even more tactical and work to redirect his head to create new openings to hit new targets such as the neck, or immediately follow up with a low-leg combative, such as a Defensive Knee or Shin Kick.

If you're to the attacker's side or for whatever reason have only one hand free, then use your free hand to gouge out the eyeball, plucking it from the socket with any free finger.

Comments • There are many ways to strike or damage your attacker's vision, and performing an Eye Gouge is one of the most effective tactics. I know that it sounds gross to attempt to scoop your attacker's eye from its socket, and it is certainly a severe level of force, but when it is a life-or-death situation, you might have to escalate the level of violence in your defense. The Eye Gouge is a technique that can be applied from many angles and many positions, and you can train to use any finger available to make contact.

Legal Ramifications • Remember this rule: You are allowed to use as much force against your attacker as he is using against you. For example, if someone is clearly not a threat to your safety, you can't gouge his eyes out and claim self-defense. Or, if you take a weapon from someone and weaken him in the process, making it so he is no longer a threat, you are not allowed to then use that weapon against him, as there is no level of force to justify the act of using the weapon once the threat has already been nullified.

ELBOW COMBATIVES

Elbows are highly effective combatives when you are close enough to use them; they work particularly well in the control range. In fact, they are my favorite combatives because they are so powerful and work from such a large variety of angles. Before I show you a series of elbow combatives, I want to take you through some effective principles of elbow combatives using our 3-Factor Combative Theory.

Target • Variety of targets, from the temple to the jaw and the sternum

Surface Area • Elbow joint, though it's important to note that you will be using slightly different areas of the elbow joint—minor differences that you will see when you practice elbow combatives later in the book. When forming or molding your elbow combative arm, make sure you always achieve these three details:

1 *Bladed Hand:* Blade your hand by simply lengthening and closing your fingers.
2 *Body Contact:* Make sure that your bladed hand is physically touching your

chest, not floating in free space; otherwise, you risk your forearm becoming the striking surface area, which diminishes the power of your combative by a large margin. Be mindful of your hand placement as you apply my muscle memory training guide, because while it's a very simple correction, it's easy to miss if you're not paying attention.

3 *Extension:* Keep your bladed hand placed as far out to your armpit as possible. For example, if you are going to elbow your attacker using your right arm, then you will want to place your right (bladed) hand as close as possible to your right armpit, instead of letting it hover farther in toward your sternum. Keeping your bladed hand out wide will elongate your arm and therefore generate more force at the striking point—the elbow joint. By doing this, it is as if you are using an arm of a body that is two to three inches taller than yours. It's details like this that allow my students who are under five foot four to be just as effective as someone who is five foot nine.

Range of Motion • Combative Twist

Combative Range • Elbows are the most effective in the Control Range. Remember that to get to the Control Range, which is your ideal range if you have no choice but to continue the fight, you'll have to first weaken the attacker with longer-range combatives, causing his structure to weaken and shorten, and granting you access to hit targets using your elbow.

Elbow Combatives How-To • To complete each elbow, first mold your weapon by blading your hand, attaching the bladed hand to your body, and rotating through the available target. Following, I list the primary angles that you should train, but when it comes to applying this combative, you will find yourself adjusting the angle automatically once you visually confirm an available target. I recommend beginning with the elbows outlined in this section and then slightly adjusting the degrees in each angle to get comfortable with your personal range of motion. Look at the photos closely to teach yourself how to mimic each combative variation.

❋ Horizontal Elbow

Target • Face, chin, jaw, side of head

Surface Area • Elbow (below elbow joint)

Range of Motion • Combative Twist

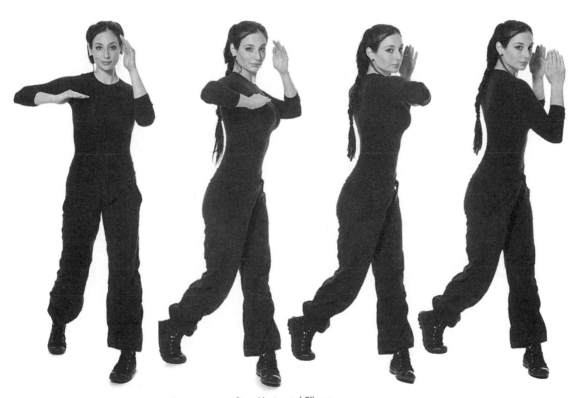

Rear Horizontal Elbow

✸ Angle Elbow

Target • Side of face, jaw, nose, temple

Surface Area • Elbow (below elbow joint)

Range of Motion • Combative Twist

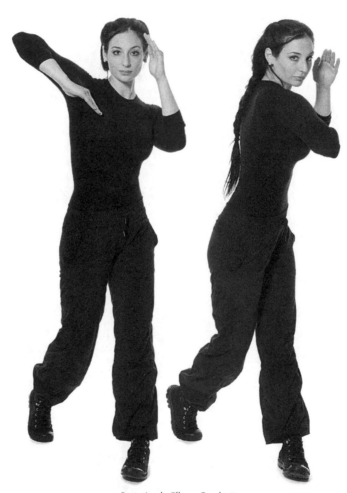

Rear Angle Elbow Combative

✻ Sky Elbow

Target • Chin, jaw

Surface Area • Elbow (below elbow joint)

Range of Motion • Combative Twist

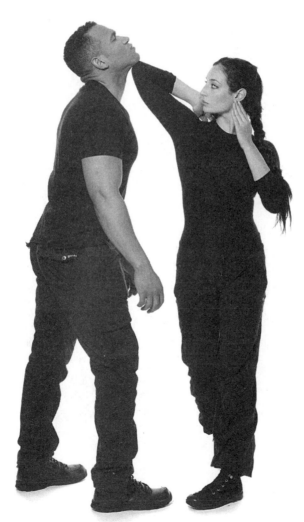

Rear Sky Elbow Combative

⊛ Hammer Elbow

Target • Back of head, back of neck, chin, side of head

Surface Area • Above the elbow joint

Range of Motion • Wind up and drop. This will require you to slightly drop your weight into your knees to drive more force.

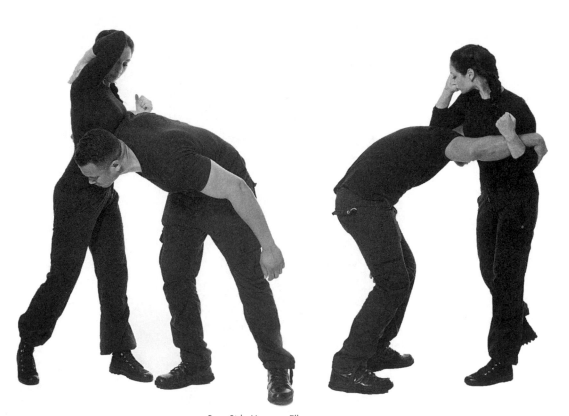

Rear-Side Hammer Elbow

Reverse Sky Elbow

Target • Chin, any center line of the body

Surface Area • Elbow (above elbow joint)

Range of Motion • Combative Twist (rear side rotation). Simply open your hips and blade your near shoulder into your attacker's body.

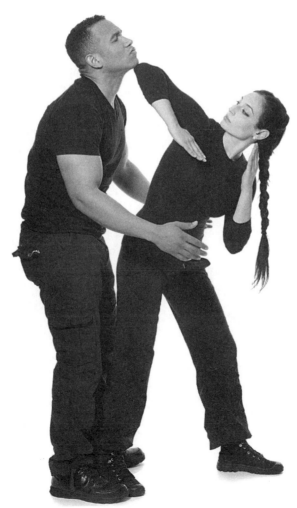

Reverse Sky Elbow

✳ Direct Rear Elbow

Target • Jaw, neck, sternum, solar plexus

Surface Area • Elbow

Range of Motion • Stepping lunge. This variation requires you to generate force and power from the distance covered by your feet. Lunge or take a fast and large step into the target to allow your elbow to drive through the target.

✳ Swinging Elbow

Target • Side of face, jaw, neck

Surface Area • Elbow (above joint)

Range of Motion • Combative Twist

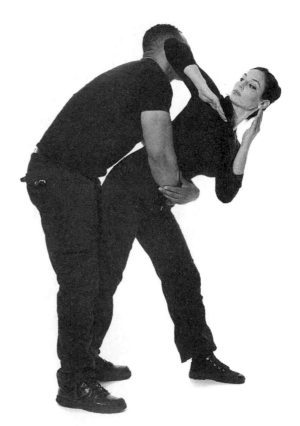

Swinging Elbow

OTHER UPPER-BODY COMBATIVES

✺ Uppercut

Target • Chin

Surface Area • Fist

Range of Motion • Combative Twist

Combative Range • Medium

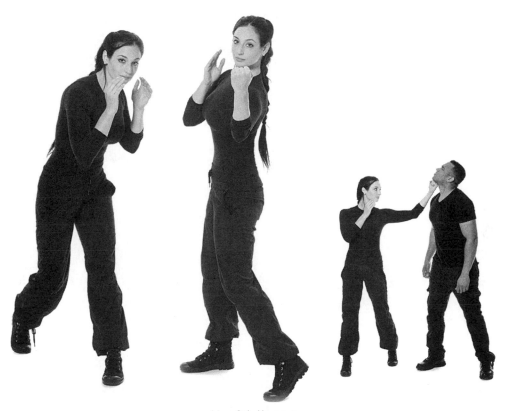

Near-Side Uppercut

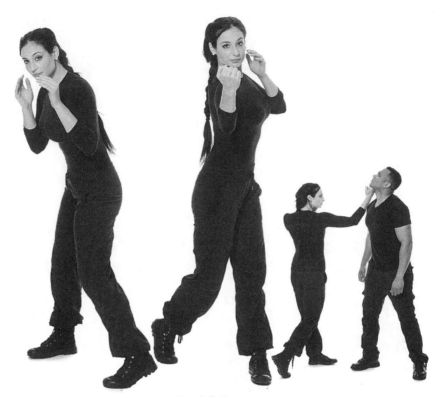

Rear-Side Uppercut

Uppercut How-To

1 Slip your body, which means to do a downward Twist initiated by the shoulder of the side you are striking with so that you overtwist in your preparation. For example, to slip to your left side from the right Survival Stance, you will drive your rear or right shoulder forward and 45 degrees downward.

2 As you slip your body, keep your arms covering your face for as long as possible to avoid telegraphing the combative (showing your preparation too early or dragging it out makes you vulnerable to a counter and gives your attacker the opportunity to adjust or prepare to counter your move). You should always train to avoid telegraphing your movements, especially when performing circular combatives, such as the Uppercut or the Hook Punch (see below), which require a longer preparation.

3 Slightly drop and then immediately swing your fist toward the ceiling, using a Combative Twist to drive the motion and surface area upward.

✤ Hook Punch

Target • Face, chin, liver, kidney

Surface Area • Fist

Range of Motion • Combative Twist

Hook Punch How-To

1 Raise your wrist to shoulder level. Bend your elbow joint 90 degrees and open up your hook position so that your fist is in line with your armpit.

2 Apply the Twist to complete the combative. Remember to keep your non-striking arm up for protection.

3 Once you've hit the target, lower your elbow immediately so that you can return to Survival Stance and avoid having your face exposed for longer than necessary.

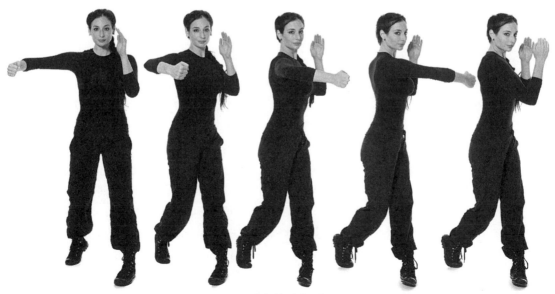

Rear-Side Hook Punch

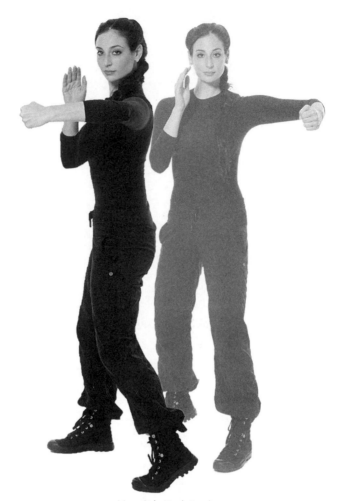

Near-Side Hook Punch

Comments • Whether you are aiming for the attacker's face or body, you want to mold your arm into a weapon by maintaining a 90-degree bend at the elbow joint and raising your forearm to be in line with your humerus bone (the bone between your shoulder and elbow joint), regardless of the intended angle. Structuring your arm this way will provide the best support to take the impact of the combative's making contact with the attacker's body.

LOWER-BODY COMBATIVES

Our legs are very powerful weapons. In this chapter I will highlight the most simple and effective kicks that can be used against an attacker. These combatives are integrated into the *Weapons of Fitness* workout routines, so pay close attention.

The primary target for the lower half on a male attacker is the groin. This vulnerable target usually results in the attacker doubling over in a forward direction, or at least flinching forward. At the very least, a groin strike will temporarily disrupt the attacker's thought process and shorten his taller frame, giving you time to come in for more upper-body and control range combatives. However, the groin won't always be an available target, so I will show you some secondary targets to aim for in those situations.

HIP THRUST: YOUR PRIMARY POWER SOURCE FOR DIRECT LOWER-BODY COMBATIVES

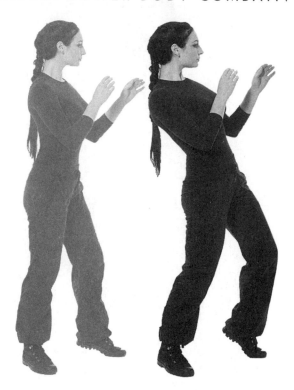

Overall, the power source for our lower-body combatives comes from the hips. Similar in nature to the twisting motion that generates power for upper-body combatives, the Hip Thrust generates power for straight lower-body combatives. Thrusting your hips is the action of driving your hips forward and slightly upward to achieve a full range of motion. As you can see in the photo above, you can test and find your full range of motion by bringing your hips forward. It is a good sign if you feel your core engaged and a slight stretch on your supporting leg's hip flexor muscle.

Hip Thrust How-To • Starting in Survival Stance, transition your weight forward while shifting your center line of support to your rear leg, or your soon-to-be supporting leg.

Near-Side Hip Thrust • To help place this in context, if you were to initiate a front kick, you would have to balance on your rear leg. However, to make the combative effective, you need to push your hips forward to increase your range of motion and power. A great way to test shifting your center line of balance is to raise your front or kicking leg off the ground to see whether you can maintain your balance on your supporting leg. Once you have found your balance on your supporting leg, return to Survival Stance and your center line of balance back to between your feet.

Rear-Side Hip Thrust • For this move, you'll follow the same principles as you did in the Near-Side Hip Thrust. Starting in Survival Stance, rotate your front, near-side leg so that your knee is turned out for balance. Continue this rotation as you drive your rear leg forward and thrust your hips forward and upward. Continue transitioning your weight forward so that you land with your previously rear leg in front. This completes your Hip Thrust motion from the rear leg. Please pay attention to the rotation and adjustment of your supporting leg that is needed to open up your hips; otherwise, you will be forced to raise your supporting heel, compromising your balance.

✳ Standing Push Kick

Target • Groin

Surface Area • Ball of the foot

Range of Motion • Hip thrust

Combative Range • Long

Comments • One of my favorite combatives, the Push Kick has the power to send someone flying back, and it can be a great tactic when you have identified a real exit (see the box on page 85) and can escape the situation.

Standing Push Kick How-To • The preparation is important, because it will help to ensure that you can extend your leg from a supported position that will also keep you on your feet in case the attacker charges in. As shown in the photo on page 84, you want to start with your standing leg slightly bent, but not bent at or past a 90-degree angle. Any greater bend at the knee joint could result in your

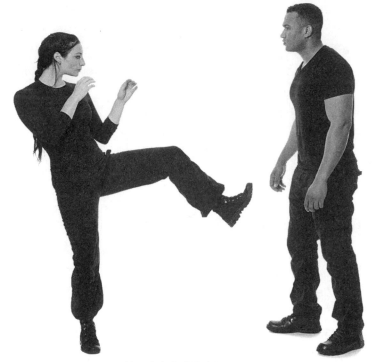

Near-Side Push Kick Preparation

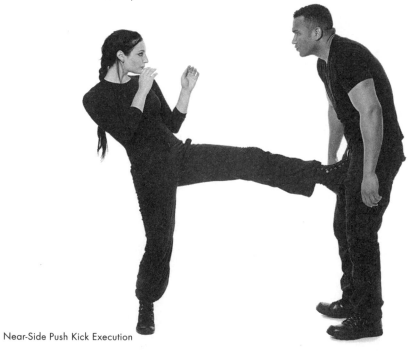

Near-Side Push Kick Execution

falling to the ground if your attacker successfully closes in to grab you or tackle you while you're trying to kick. To fully execute the kick, drive the ball of your foot through the target with as much power as possible using the Hip Thrust. Once you've made contact, continue to transition your body weight forward and then bring your foot back to the Survival Stance as fast as possible to continue your defense.

Ground Survival Position

Before I show you how to apply the Push Kick from the ground range, I want to show you my Ground Survival Position. This is the position I get into the second I find myself on my back: I brace my legs to create a gate across my body. I drive one knee across to use that leg's shinbone as the gate, and I flex my other leg's foot so that I have the heel ready to use as a reference point on the attacker's body. By immediately bracing, I am ready to use the power of my legs against

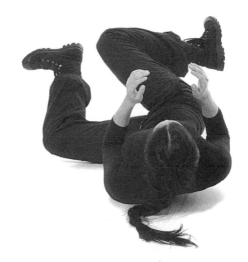

an attacker trying to gain access in between my legs, and I am ready to kick and and earn the ability to safely return to my feet—once the threat is no longer active. When it comes to engaging in Defensive Ground Push Kicks from this position, I simply need to rotate my braced knee into my chest, while I simultaneously plant my non-kicking leg's foot on the ground to support the kicking leg, to engage in any angled Ground Push Kick. I can also break the angle from this position in case the attacker is circling me. As far as my arm position, I keep the guarded upper-body position from Survival Stance so that I have a central point to operate and adapt from. Ultimately, my leg position creates a difficult barrier for an attacker to break through and gives me the flexibility to transition into any lower-body movement necessary for survival, while my upper body is centered and ready to work.

✳ Ground Push Kick

Target • Groin, knee, face

Surface Area • Ball of the foot or heel to the groin, heel to the face and heel to the knee. Whether you are on your feet or your back, the ball of the foot is a great

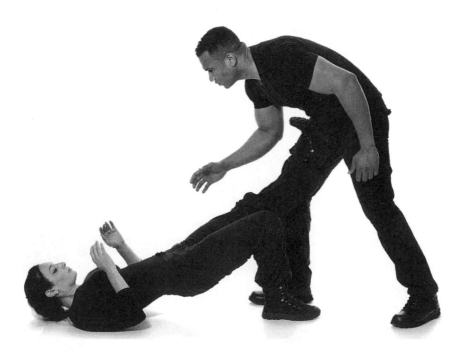

surface area to train as a default reaction because it works for both ranges. The heel is also a great surface area to use when you are on the ground, as it can easily make contact with your primary target points.

Range of Motion • Hip Thrust

Combative Range • Ground

Ground Push Kick How-To • You will apply the same leg preparation position as you did before extending for the Standing Push Kick. Have the surface area ready and hit the target by thrusting your hips to the sky as you fully extend the leg into the target. A great way to practice generating this power source is to perform basic pelvis raises to the ceiling.

Weapons of Fitness **Benefit** • This is a great exercise for strengthening your core and your glutes.

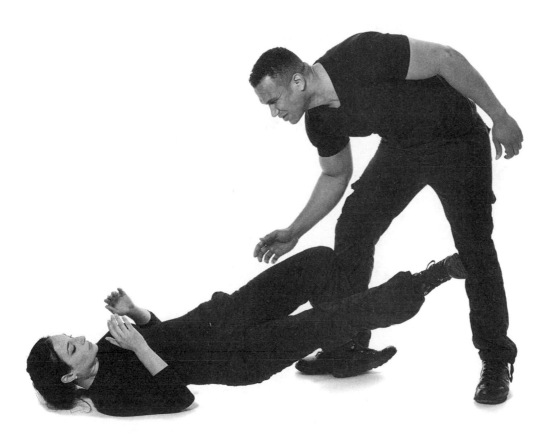

✳ Snap Kick

Target • Groin

Surface Area • Top of toes

Range of Motion • Forward Hip Thrust

Combative Range • Long Range

Snap Kick How-To • To fully execute the Snap Kick, drive the top of your toes through the target with as much power as possible using the Hip Thrust. Once you have made contact, continue to transition your body weight forward, and then bring your foot back into the Survival Stance as fast as possible to continue your defense.

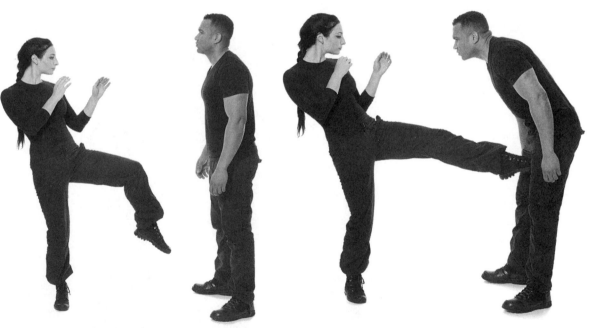

Near-Side Snap Kick Preparation   Near-Side Snap Kick

Comments • Over time, making the decision to use a certain combative and to try for power or speed will become second nature and your instincts will be guided toward focusing on the next move, instead of reacting and hoping for certain outcomes. So here is the general rule when it comes to power versus speed: Use speed combatives when you want to close in on the attacker's body to get to the control range. Use your power combatives when you want to drive the attacker's body as far away as possible so you can escape—or if you have control of the body and want to deliver as many combatives as you can.

Power vs. Speed

AS YOU TRANSITION BACK TO YOUR FEET FROM THE GROUND PUSH KICK, YOU can strategically control certain elements and outcomes of your combatives. I realized this when I was applying the Push Kick into scenario training drills. When I delivered as much power as possible behind a Push Kick, it worked only when I had an escape or a real exit; when I practiced it in a closed environment without an exit, it actually made it much more difficult to close in for a Control Hold (see page 106) or to successfully follow up and make contact with more combatives. It was then that I realized that combatives can be executed with either power as the primary focus (in which case the Push Kick would force the attacker away from my body, granting me the chance to escape) or speed as the primary focus (in which case the Snap Kick would still disrupt the attacker's thought process but not push the attacker away). For closed environments without an obvious exit, I began to modify the Push Kick by shifting my focus to speed and using the top of my foot to target the groin. This resulted in the attacker hunching over and granting me access to his head, leading to the creation of the Snap Kick.

✹ Combative Knee

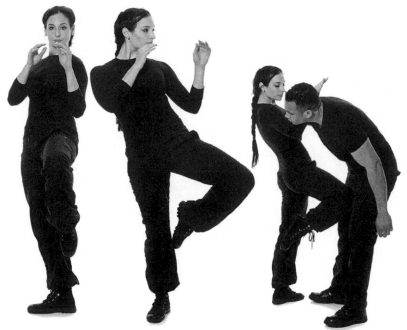

Near-Side Combative Knee   Rear-Side Combative Knee

Target • Groin (primary), face, chest

Surface Area • Kneecap

Range of Motion • Hip Thrust

Combative Range • Control Range

Combative Knee How-To • Raise your knee sharply in the path of the identified target. Make sure that you immediately tuck your foot back so that it doesn't get in the path of your knee. As you raise your knee, simultaneously do a Hip Thrust to drive the surface area into the target.

Comments • The Combative Knee is one of the most effective close-range lower-body moves. This is a great power combative when you are close and temporarily controlling the attacker, say, with one arm wrapped around his arm, and can control his physical reaction to the impact. For example, once you get into control range and can temporarily control your attacker's body via a hook control position with your arm over his arm, you can deliver a powerful knee combative to the groin—while still maintaining control. When you perform the Combative Knee, you use your kneecap to make contact with your attacker. The first and primary target should be the attacker's groin, as striking his groin at that range and having him bend over in pain will grant you immediate and direct access to multiple targets and more opportunities to counterstrike. Other areas to target include the face and the chest, which, if he is bent over, will be open and available. If you have the opportunity to deliver the Combative Knee, use it over and over again in quick succession until his structure is weakened or until another and better combative or opportunity arises to neutralize the attack, such as a Shin Kick (which I personally use) or a Downward Elbow Combative.

✷ Shin Kick

Target • Groin

Surface Area • Shin

Range of Motion • Forward Hip Thrust

Combative Range • Medium/Control Range

Shin Kick How-To • Extend and firmly straighten your leg to drive your shinbone in between and upward through your attacker's body. The motion consists of raising your shin between the attacker's legs and driving the bone directly upward to the center of his body.

Comments • This is a target-specific strike, aimed directly for the groin. The anterior surface area of the shin targets right underneath the attacker's groin. This is great to use either as a follow-up or in between several Combative Knees.

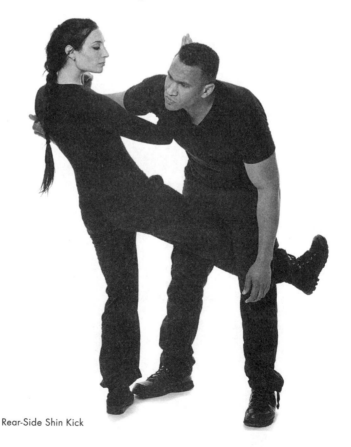

Rear-Side Shin Kick

✳ Side Kick

Target • Knee, torso, groin

Surface Area • Heel of the foot for the groin, knee, and torso; ball of the foot for the groin

Range of Motion • Twisted lateral extension. To help clarify, the twisted lateral extension means that you will be rotating one side of your body against the direction of your combative. This is done by simultaneously driving your near shoulder and hipbone in the opposite direction of your intended target.

Combative Range • Long

Comments • The Side Kick is the longest-range kick you have when you are measuring the length of space from your head and chest to the attacker's body. The

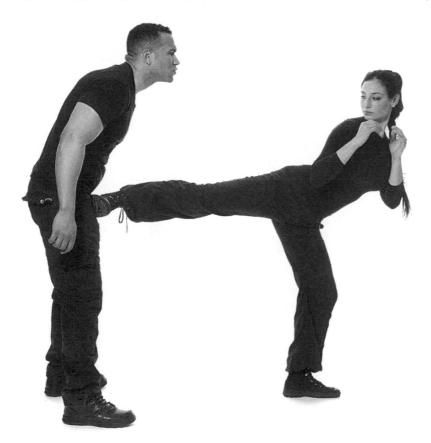

Side Kick uses the hard bone of the heel of the lead foot to make contact with the target. This is effective against unarmed attackers, to maintain space, and also against edged weapons, as it allows your body to be as far away from the blade as possible while still engaging in a defensive combative.

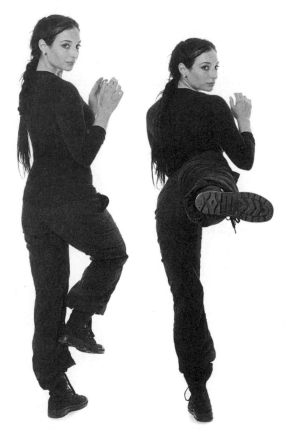

Side Kick Preparation and Execution

Side Kick How-To

1 Whether you begin facing your attacker or are already positioned in the side stance, you can set up the angle for a twisted lateral extension by raising your knee and flexing your foot while imagining that you are showing one back jean pocket to your attacker (as a helpful visual of what the preparation position looks like). Based on this angle, you will continuously extend the striking leg by turning the inside of the foot so that it is parallel to the ground. Your base leg will open by rotating on the ball of the foot. You can choose to keep your body more upright or lean forward so that your torso is almost parallel to the ground.

2 Raise your knee to the level of your hips to set up the angle for the Side Kick, then drive the bottom of your foot out forcefully to make contact via your heel with the attacker's groin, knee, or torso. Immediately return to Survival Stance.

3 If you're standing to the side of your attacker, you're in a great position to bring him to his knees simply by side-kicking the back outer corner of his knee, forcing the knee to buckle and your attacker to fall. (See the next page.)

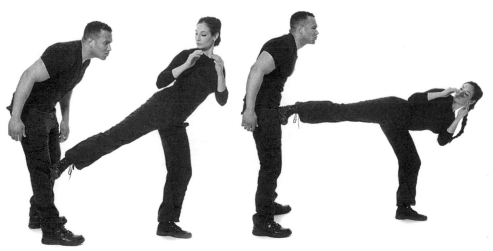

Low Side Kick   Extended Side Kick

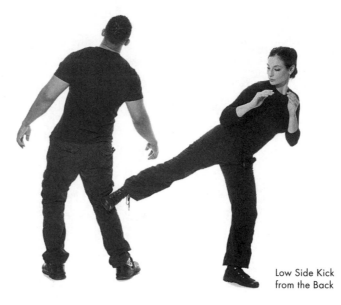

Low Side Kick
from the Back

✳ Ground Side Kick

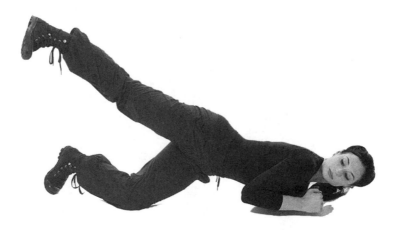

Target · Knee, groin

Surface Area · Heel or ball of foot

Range of Motion · Twisted lateral extension

Combative Range · Ground

Ground Side Kick How-To

1   Starting on your back with your legs fully extended, shift your body to one side so you can set up your side kick on the ground. Bring your arms into Survival Stance position so that you are protected.

2   Transfer your weight onto your shoulder as you raise your hips off the ground. This will create an opening between your body and the floor, allowing you to slide your knee upward to serve as your supporting leg when you initiate the side kick.

3   As you raise your hips in step 2, simultaneously bring your kicking leg's knee in toward your chest, similar to the preparation outlined in the stand-up Side Kick.

4   Rotate your near shoulder to the ground as you extend the heel of your kicking leg into your target. This cross motion will allow you to drive your heel into any target level (as it is outlined by height).

5   Once you have made contact with your target, immediately return your leg to the starting position.

Comments • This is an extremely powerful ground-based combative. As you apply the same principle of generating force using the twisted lateral extension, you will see that you can successfully target the attacker's knee if he is standing over you. I have also used the ball of my foot as the surface area when I was within range to make contact with the groin. Both are effective, and once you identify an open target, you will watch your body morph with the right muscle memory to use the correct surface area—but this happens only when you drive your training to focus on adaptive concepts like recognizing the target first. For this reason alone, train to do both variations.

✴ **Rear Kick**

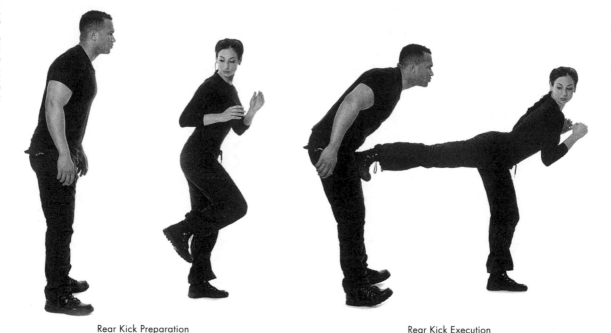

Rear Kick Preparation   Rear Kick Execution

Target • Groin or midsection

Surface Area • Heel

Range of Motion • Chest dip

Combative Range • Long

Rear Kick How-To • Flex your foot and raise your knee to your chest. The preparation for the Rear Kick is similar to that for the Side Kick; however, instead of imagining you are showing the attacker one jean pocket, position yourself as if you are showing him both jean pockets. Extend your heel into the target and achieve your full range of motion by bringing your chest slightly forward so you can raise your leg.

Comments • The Rear Kick is a great option if you become aware of someone behind you, or if you are facing multiple attackers. This kick is very similar to the Side Kick, as it requires you to keep your chest and hips facing the ground as you extend your heel out and immediately bring it back.

✹ Roundhouse Kick

Target • Knee, torso

Surface Area • Shin

Range of Motion • Hip swing

Combative Range • Medium

Roundhouse Kick How-To

1 Begin by raising your knee to the level of the open target (i.e., your attacker's knee with a low kick or his torso with a high kick).

2 Once you reach the level you're aiming for, rotate your hips toward the target and continue driving your hips through so that they pass the target. This will cause your shinbone to align with the target and make contact.

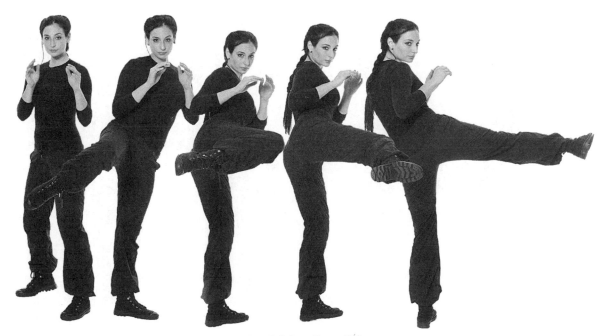

Rear-Side Roundhouse Kick

3 Even though you are training to drive your shin through the target, once you make contact with the attacker's body, you will bounce back, so make sure that you bounce back into Survival Position.

Comments • The advantage in implementing Straight Kicks, such as the Push Kick or Snap Kick, is that the surface area is delivered to the target as soon as possible, because the direct path is the shortest path, and therefore the quickest. However, I do endorse Roundhouse Kicks as a secondary combative to learn in case you recognize an opening and would like to strategically break down your attacker's structure or set up a following combative. Practice aiming for both the knee and the torso.

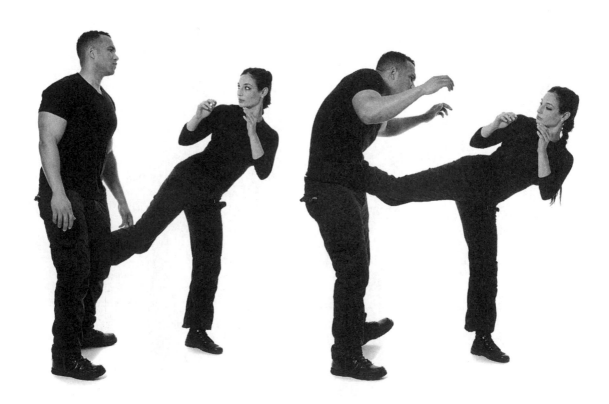

✳ Roundhouse Knee

Target • Groin

Surface Area • Kneecap

Range of Motion • Hip Swing

Combative Range • Medium

Roundhouse Knee How-To

1. Raise your knee to the level of the target, but for this variation, flare your knee outward, which will also open up your hips, giving you the preparation distance required to help generate force once you swing the hips through.

2. To make contact, drive your hips around and through the target by using your rear hip to lead and travel through the horizontal path.

Comments • This is a great variation to the direct Defensive Knee—when you are launching the knee from a Control Hold, which will be highlighted in the next chapter. Training to do the Roundhouse Knee will show you that you can adapt to an attacker's unpredictable reactions with the same combative to make sure you don't miss the target.

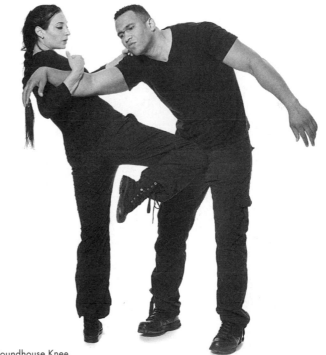

Roundhouse Knee

DRILL: FINDING YOUR FORMULA

Objective • Part of making the Soteria Method work for you includes identifying the combatives that work best for you, as well as developing a single series of combatives that will successfully transition you through the striking ranges. I recommend training so that a combination of combatives at different ranges becomes second nature as your survival response—in case you ever need to use it. For example, if you have had a couple of drinks and you are faced with a threat, you should be able to perform the combination either offensively or defensively. Personally, I learned that by having a trained formula to default to under stress would help me overcome the mental and physical freeze when my mind would recognize the need to engage defensively in combatives.

Breaking Down Your Formula

To create a formula of combatives that will transition you from long range to control range as quickly as possible, select one combative in each range that flows from the near to the rear side and stick to a combination that works for you. Just remember, we want to earn the right and ultimately the safety to get into the control range. Getting to the control range or gaining control of the attacker's head means that you have done everything possible to physically and mentally weaken the attacker and to disrupt his thought process. At this stage, you can then control him with less resistance and focus on neutralizing the situation.

Here's an example of a combative flow that I like: Near-Side Snap Kick | Near-Side Finger Flick | Rear-Side Shin Kick | New Near-Side Elbow. "New Near-Side" refers to the fact that as you transition from the Rear-Side Shin Kick into your next combative, you will be alternating your Survival Stance to put your other leg in front, giving you a new near side—which is why you want to make sure that you are training and building up the Survival Stance on both sides.

REGARDLESS OF THE SPECIFIC COMBATIVES you select for a series, the formula is quite versatile, as it can be applied to the following scenarios:

1 When you first confirm that someone has threatened your safety, but he hasn't acted yet.

2 When an attacker is already in motion, but you are within kicking range (long range).

3 When the attacker is already within striking range (medium range).

4 When the attacker is within your personal circle (medium range/control range).

5 When you might not be in your best state (e.g., you have had some wine at a party and are caught by surprise by the attack) and you have to defend yourself.

DEFENDING YOURSELF

Turning your body into a weapon and learning to use combatives to defend yourself is only one part of the Soteria Method. I'm now going to introduce the Soteria Method Survival Pyramid, a four-phase response process that I formed to simplify tactics in my mind while being armed to adapt to the dynamics of a real-life situation. In this chapter, I will highlight basic defenses as shown in this pyramid to give you an insight on the whole method as it relates to self-defense against an attack. I will also show you the blocks and control holds that you will use most often when you face any kind of attack. These will be your trained default reactions to ensure that you don't overthink or add time onto your RACE Reaction. Later in the chapter, I'll explain how you can work these into a flow with your combatives to ultimately gain the right to strike—and to survive.

SOTERIA METHOD SURVIVAL PYRAMID

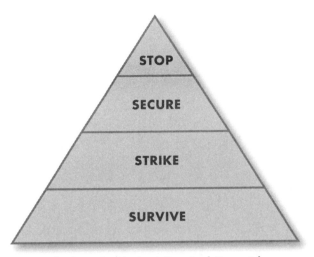

The Soteria Method Survival Pyramid

The four phases of the Soteria Method Survival Pyramid are Stop, Secure, Strike, and Survive. These four clear phases will become your milestones in completing your defense from start to finish. Once you become familiar with this process, you will begin to experience a trained reaction that is both efficient and adaptable to the uncertainties and ever-changing variables of the street, including attackers' different levels of pain tolerance and different physical profiles, and additional challenges such as multiple attackers. Let's go over each phase in more detail.

Phase 1: Stop

You must first stop and intercept the initial attack, whatever it may be. You will learn reactions specific to certain attacks later in this chapter, allowing you to retain and utilize simplified concepts under pressure.

I designed the Stop phase to be as simple as possible so that you can create automatic "default defense reactions." The second you recognize a threat or find yourself being attacked, you need to intercept and stop the attack from getting worse. In the best-case scenario, this means that that you evade or escape the attack or physically remove yourself from the attacker's path. However, the reality is that you might recognize the attack only after it has begun, and escaping might not be an immediate option. For this reason, I'm also giving you an example of a single defensive move called Blocking, which can be applied to multiple attacks or variations of the same attack. The point here is that you can simplify what you retain both mentally and physically as a defense so that it comes to your aid immediately.

Active vs. Static Attacks

REMEMBER, SIMPLICITY IS SURVIVAL. WHEN I WAS LOOKING FOR COMMON DE-nominators while forming my pyramid, I categorized attacks based on whether they were "active" or "static." An active attack means one that is in motion—leaving you with your trained or natural reflexes to save you in the initial Stop phase of defense. Examples of an active attack include slashes, punches, and the use of impact weapons, such as swinging a bat. A static attack, on the other hand, refers to one that has a static reference point, including a choke hold, a grab, and a knife or gun threat. It is important to train for an attack in both of these categories to help you tactically assess the attack more efficiently. Building your skills in these categories will help you complete Phase 2 (Analyze) of the RACE Reaction in a much more efficient and effective way.

Phase 2: Secure

Once you have intercepted the original threat or attack, you should attempt to escape if you can. However, if you are in a closed environment without an easy escape, you will have to close in and secure the attacker. This brings us to the Control Hold, which is the ultimate goal in Phase 2. The two hook positions that I work from are the Temporary Under Hook Control Hold and the Temporary Over-Hook Control Hold. Both are designed to secure the active arm of the attacker. Depending on the actions you completed in the Stop phase, you will transition into whatever Control Hold is available. From the mechanical perspective, the Control Holds allow you to secure the attacker's arm by trapping him close to your

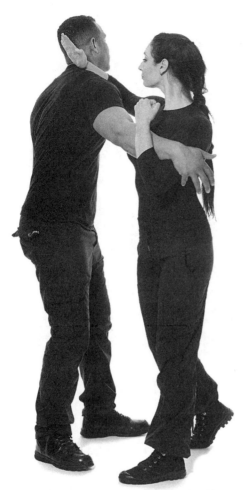 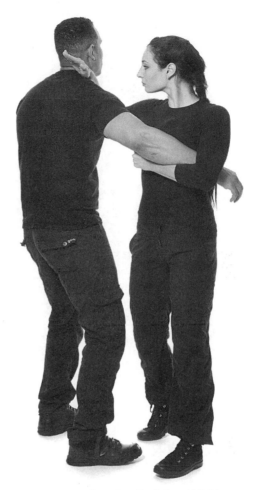

Temporary Front Under-Hook Control Hold   Temporary Front Over-Hook Control Hold

body, which will position you to perform knee and shin kick combatives. Please note that you might be able to get to this phase after two or three combatives designed to disrupt his thought process during the Stop phase.

The second you get your attacker into a Control Hold, you must immediately transition into Phase 3 to capitalize on the control before you lose contact—because you have to assume that at some point you will lose contact, as your attacker struggles to release himself from your grip. Here I'll break down the Control Holds and show you how you can secure control, even temporarily.

Control Hold Tips: As you can see in the images above, the Control Hold is

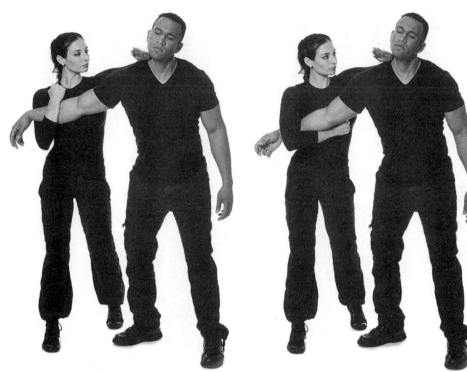

Temporary Back Under-Hook Control Hold   Temporary Back Over-Hook Control Hold

simple and highly effective, as long as you commit to the details. First, whether you are hooking over or under the attacker's arm, make sure that you are squeezing your forearm to your bicep, even if that means angling your arm to close the gap. The second gap that you need to close is any distance between your body and the attacker's arm. This is important, because by gluing your body to his arm, you immediately make it harder for him to retract and resist. Your near arm should be bladed, and you can use your forearm to keep his body upright. Finally, your feet should be in Survival Stance, helping you maintain your balance and getting you ready for Phase 3—weakening the attacker with combatives.

Phase 3: Strike

As the name explains, here's where you work to break down the attacker's structure. I recommend training a default reaction of three Combative Knees, and from

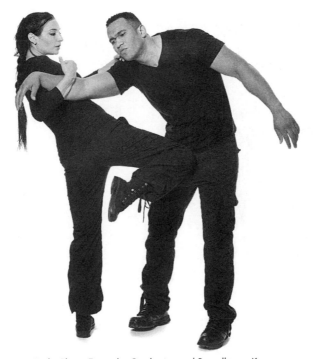

Strike Phase Example: Combative and Roundhouse Knee

there you can add on any variations as necessary; I personally like to follow up with a Shin Kick. The common reaction from the knee to the groin is for the attacker to at least hunch over. If he is on drugs or has a high tolerance for pain, you will immediately feel and recognize the resistance in his body, meaning you will need to engage in more severe combatives such as the Eye Gouge. I also recommend preparing to look for secondary targets, such as the back of the attacker's knee. If you side-kicked him in the back of the knee from the control position, he would likely drop to his knees, thus providing you with easier and more direct access to his face. For those of you who are short in stature, I recommend following your Combative Knee with a Side Kick to the back of the knee as a primary combative. Above, I've used the Roundhouse Knee to show you an example of the three knee moves you can use during this phase. When you execute this move, continue to reestablish your Survival Stance, but also drive your stance forward to add additional force and power.

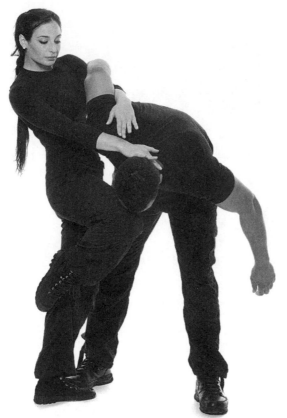

Survive Phase Example:
Combative Knee Targeting the Face

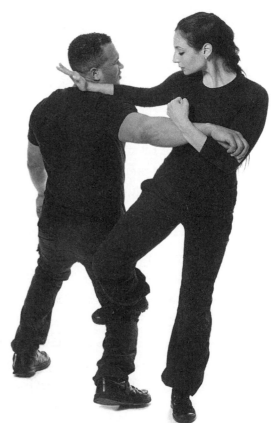

Survive Phase Example:
Low Side Kick to the Back of the Knee

Phase 4: Survive

This is where you need to neutralize and end the attack. Continuing on from Phase 3, if the attacker is hunched over from your combatives, then you can perform additional knees to his face, do a Side Kick to the back of his leg, and elbow him. If he wasn't reactive in Phase 3, you can either do a Side Kick to the back corner of his knee to bring him down to his knees and then go for an Eye Gouge (assuming this amount of force is justified by his previous actions), perform an upper-body combative such as an elbow, or strike and squeeze his Adam's apple—simply grab his Adam's apple like an egg and squeeze it with your hand as you simultaneously complete the action of attempting to rip it out of his neck.

If you are facing an unarmed attack without a clear real exit, you need to make sure he is down on the ground and neutralized before you attempt to escape. If you are facing an armed attacker, make sure that you have disarmed him and that he is down and neutralized. (Note: I am not highlighting weapon defense in this book, but the Soteria Method Survival Pyramid also applies to weapon defense.) If you are facing an attack while on the ground, make sure you can get back up on your feet safely; I outline how to safely get up from the ground later in this chapter (see "Ground-Range Choking"). When you have confirmed that your attacker is no longer a threat, never give up your guard, even in the escape, because you never know if the attacker will be able to recover and reattack or if there is an accomplice. Don't assume anything until you can confirm that you are safe.

DEFENSIVE MOVES

Blocking

As you learned in Phase 1 of the pyramid, the first thing you need to accomplish is to stop the attack. To that end, I'm going to teach you a basic block. Against an active attack, no matter whether it's in the form of a punch, an attempted grab, or even a knife attack, the Block defense will stop the attacker's hand from making contact with your face from any angle.

Practice this blocking position over and over, especially coming into it from various positions, so that you'll have one immediate response that works in any

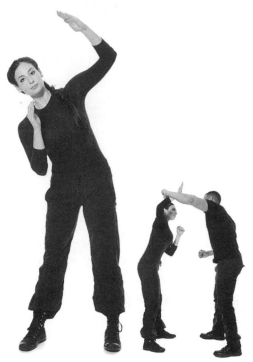

Defensive Upper-Body Blocks

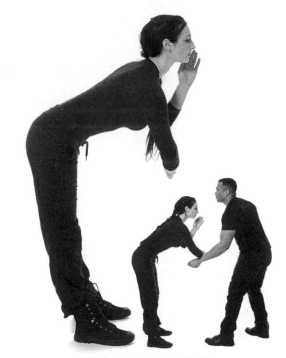

Defensive Lower-Body Blocks

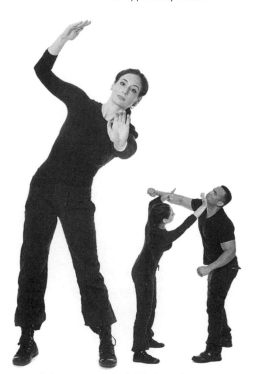

Defensive Upper-Body Blocks and Counter

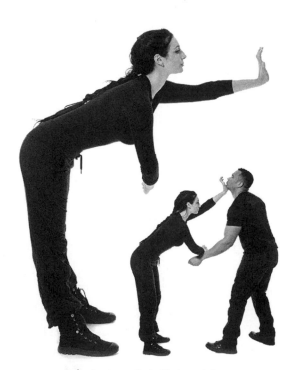

Defensive Lower-Body Blocks and Counter

scenario. Creating a common denominator defense is a key concept and strategy in the Soteria Method, because by simplifying your movements, you ensure that no matter what the attacker has in his hand, you will be able to stop and intercept an attack from the most vulnerable position or moment, and work your way through the pyramid to escape to safety.

Blocking a Hook Punch

The block works against both circular and direct active attacks. Regardless of the angle, I work with one arm position to create a consistent shield. To block the classic Hook Punch, which uses a circular angle, I train my body to lean away from the threat that I can see in my peripheral vision. I have trained to use three basic body movements: lean to the left, lean to the right, and drive my hips back. I make sure that the inside of my wrist is not exposed, in case the attacker is holding an edged weapon. I train myself to be mindful of keeping a certain distance between the forearm of my blocking arm and my head or body, depending on whether the attack is aimed above my sternum or below my sternum. With practice, this distance will become something your mind calculates automatically, and the calculation goes faster if you are using your peripheral vision. It is your responsibility to train this position consistently, because if you aren't able to block, you won't be able to transition into the next phase—or at least you will be compromised and it will be tougher to do so.

As you can see in the images on the previous page, I have included a Block variation with a counterstrike, which means I go directly from a defensive Block to an offensive combative. I want you to first train the Block to achieve the muscle memory before adding on the counter, because the Block is what will save you. If you make the counterstrike the primary focus, you run the risk of not training the Block as thoroughly, and that is something you can't afford to take a chance on. Once you have mastered the Block and are looking to add a counter, the Palm Strike is a great option, as it should accomplish the disruption in the attacker's thought process that allows you to safely transition into Phase 2, securing the body.

Defensive Block How-To

When it comes to training and developing a strong blocking arm position, I keep it simple. Reference these factors to build up a consistent shield with your arm:

1 *Hand:* Make sure you keep your hand bladed by squeezing your fingers together. This is important because when you use the length of your forearm to block, the full extension of your hand will add on a couple of inches and magnify your ability to block a fast-incoming swing.

2 *Elbow Joint:* Maintain a 90-degree bend at your elbow joint. This is crucial to ensuring that you allow your forearm to block the attack. If you bend your elbow at a degree greater than 90 degrees, you will lose the amount of space between your arm and body. On the other hand, if you maintain a bend in your elbow joint that is less than 90 degrees, you will create a "slide," because once the impact of the attack makes contact with your arm, it will slide down to your body, and that is a problem you cannot afford—especially if the attacker is armed with an edged weapon.

3 *Body Movement:* As the objective of the Block is to stop an attack and maintain distance between your arm and your body, moving your body will play a significant part in ensuring that a protected space is created as quickly and efficiently as possible. For upper-body attacks, or attacks that take place above the sternum, the body movement involves leaning your body to the right or the left—away from the side that the attack is coming in from. When it comes to an attack aimed below your sternum, the movement simply involves you driving your hips backward. Finally, if the attack is directly in front of you, the body motion is to simultaneously lean and blade your body.

4 *Putting It All Together:* In order to effectively block, train your arm position simultaneously with your body movement to develop a consistent position as you rework your reflexive response. You will then begin to notice that as your body and arm engage in the correct movements, your mind will have the ability to respond to the angle of the attack detected by your peripheral vision.

I train a primary upper-body block against a circular attack, a primary lower-body block against a lower circular attack, and a single block to redirect a direct strike aimed for the center of my body. I train three primary blocks because it allows my mind to adapt those blocks to the specific angles that are unique from one attack to another.

APPLYING THE SOTERIA METHOD SURVIVAL PYRAMID
Choke-Hold Release, Front and Side

Let's work through our defensive reactions using the Soteria Method Survival Pyramid to see how simple self-defense can be. Here's how to release yourself from a front or a side choke hold.

If you are being choked around the neck, you need to release the attacker's grip as quickly as possible. The longer your airway is restricted, the better your chance of falling unconscious—which is what your attacker wants. To break the choke

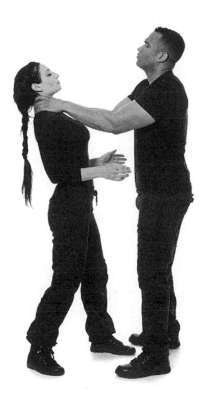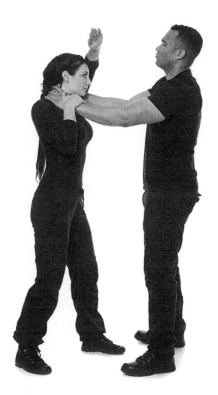

hold, create a lock around his hands, release the lock using the Combative Twist you learned in Chapter 5, and immediately launch a counterattack to disrupt his thought process so that you can transition into the next phase of defense. Follow the instructions outlined below for each phase of the pyramid to stop and release his grip.

Stop: To stop the attack, you need to release yourself from the attacker's choke grip. Draw your near-side arm (the one closest to your attacker) over your head, creating a tight lock between your bicep and your ear and trapping your attacker's hand and wrist in that space. Simultaneously, use your rear-side hand

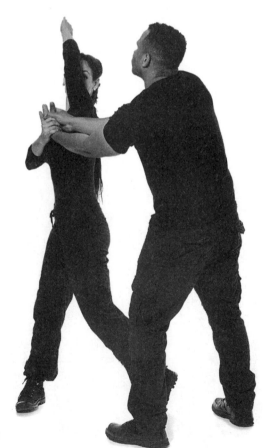

Using the Combative Twist
to Release a Choke Hold

(the one farthest from your attacker) to grab the outside of your attacker's thumb (in between the thumb and wrist). For the lock to be successful, you have to eliminate the space between your bicep and ear.

Now it's time for the Twist. Apply the same twisting motion that you learned for your upper-body combatives, driving through the turn from your core with explosive force. Keep an eye on your attacker as you move, and do not expose your back to him. As you twist, simultaneously pluck the attacker's other hand off the other side of your neck by applying sudden force and flaring the inside of his palm out as you pull it away from yourself—but keep hold of it.

Pull your attacker's body into you as you release the choke hold by keeping his plucked hand close to your chest. This will temporarily lock his arms in place, giving you control of the situation and space to execute a counterattack. To complete the first phase, capitalize on the sudden release with a quick Back Hammer Fist or Side Elbow. See the photos below to view both the Back Hammer Fist and the Side Elbow.

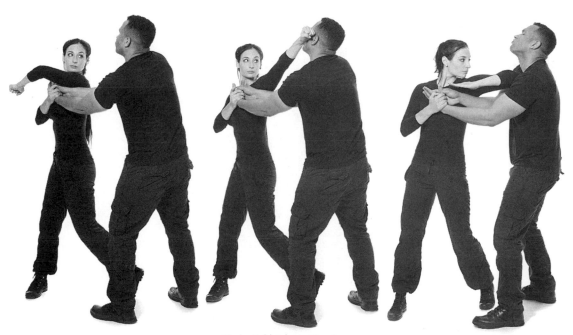

Choke-Hold Release Counters

Secure: To execute the Control Hold, make sure that you always take a large step to the side of his body to remove yourself from his countering planes. The most natural Control Hold to obtain from the choke release is the Under Hook Control Hold. If you are short, you can modify the Control Hold by placing your close arm on his bicep or by grabbing his jacket sleeve to close the gap between your body and his arm. (See the "Phase 2: Secure" section on page 106 to review the Control Holds, if needed.)

Strike: To capitalize on your temporary control hold, immediately engage in multiple combatives. I recommend starting with Combative Knees.

Survive: Use multiple combatives until the attacker is down and no longer a threat, allowing you to escape safely. (See the "Phase 4: Survive" pyramid section on page 111 to review the combatives, if needed.)

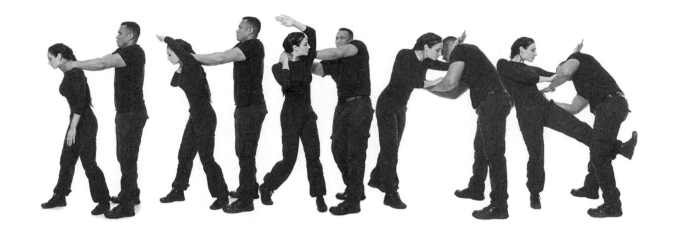

Choke-Hold Release, Rear Push

Now let's look at applying the pyramid phases—Stop, Secure, Strike, Survive—against a choke hold from the rear.

When you're being choked from the rear, you immediately need to get into Survival Stance to maintain your balance and avoid getting pushed to the ground. You will find that you'll automatically transition into one side of your Survival Stance. Depending on which foot is forward from your natural Survival Stance, you will be raising the bicep of your near-side arm to make contact with the side of your face. This ensures that you are closing the gap between your arm and body, resulting in the tightest grip possible. Remember, the tighter the lock you create around the attacker's grip, the more effective the release will be when you twist to release the choke hold. Once you create this lock, twist the body toward his locking arm to release his grip, and immediately put your hands on his arm, so that you can counter by using a Shin Kick. From here, you will then be able to pick up the rest of your defense as you work your way down the pyramid.

Choke-Hold Release, Rear Pull

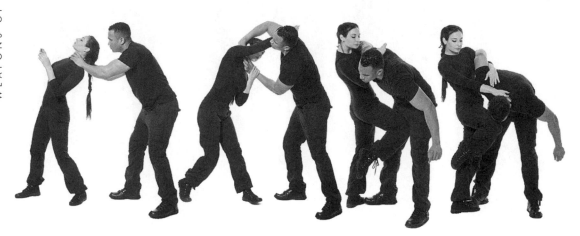

Stop: To stop a pulling choke from the rear, your body will automatically attempt to stay on your feet, and you will be able to do so by getting into Survival Stance. When this happens at full speed, you will feel an extreme pull—like your back is bending in half. Instead of trying to pull your head and torso back to an upright position, which will only cut off your air supply more quickly, go with the attacker's pull by turning into your rear leg and driving the top of your head into his sternum. Simultaneously place your near-side hand over his hand to pluck it off your body as you twist. Immediately twisting will help you make the transition so that you are no longer giving him access to your back. By going with the pull and turning into him, you gain the opportunity to set up a diagonal reach across his body so you can transition into Phase 2.

Secure: As you can see in the image above, I am transitioning toward a classic Under-Hook Control Hold, and the diagonal reach from Phase 1 allows me to immediately place my forearm across his neck as a reference point.

Strike: Immediately go into combatives, with three Combative Knees and follow-up moves.

Survive: Continue to use multiple combatives until the attacker is down and no longer a threat, allowing you to escape safely.

Hair-Grab Release, Rear Pull

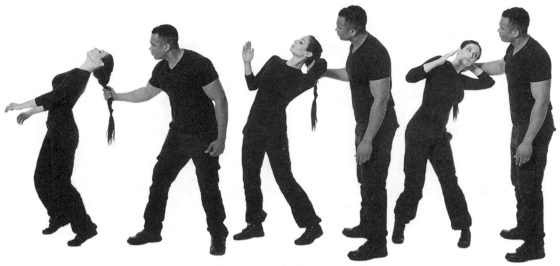

Stop Phase: Hair-Grab Release, Rear Pull

If someone is holding your hair, that person has a lot of power over your entire body. When I was testing this defense, it felt very personal, because my attacker had used this hold on me, and I know firsthand how much control it gave him. As I trained in self-defense, I learned that to stop the pull, either I had to grab higher than the grip my attacker had—similar to what I do when I am trying to brush out my hair—or I had to hold on to his hand to prevent him from pulling more hair and getting my body in a more compromising position.

My experience testing this defense was actually the event that prompted my discovery of the positive-angle approach to self-defense: No matter how bad a situation feels, you can uncover a positive that can work to your advantage. In the case of the hair grab, your advantages are that your attacker has already invited you into the Control Range, that he has given up one of his personal combative weapons by using one hand to hold you, and that you know he's not holding a weapon in that hand.

Stop: To stop the hair pull, simply grab on to the top of his hand if he has a deep grip, or grab above his grip if there is space to do so on your hair. Start by grabbing the top of your own head and moving your hand down till it's just above or on top of his hand.

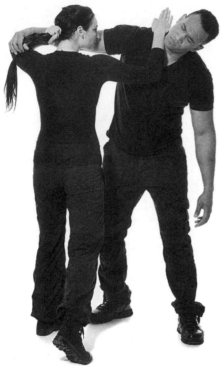

Secure Phase: Hair-Grab Release, Rear Pull

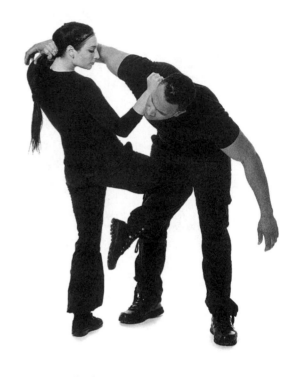

Strike Phase: Hair-Grab Release, Rear Pull

Secure: For a modified Under Hook Control, follow the Control Hold principles. Close in so that your body touches the center of the attacker's arm. Blade your hand across his neck, ready to grab on to clothing if you need to. Keep your feet and legs in Survival Stance, ready to knee and weaken him. The only difference between this and a standard Under Hook Control is that your hand remains on his hand.

Strike: Immediately go into combatives, with three Combative Knees and combative follow-ups.

Survive: Continue to use multiple combatives until the attacker is down and no longer a threat, allowing you to escape safely.

Hair-Grab Release, Front

I'll keep this explanation simple so that you can test the concepts I outlined above and see the simplicity of the pyramid.

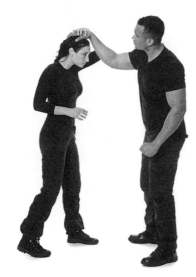

Stop Phase: Hair-Grab Release, Front Pull

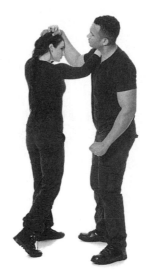

Secure Phase: Hair-Grab Release, Front Pull

Stop: Place your hand on his hand to prevent him from continuing to control your body.

Secure: Do a modified Control Hold by closing your chest into his arms and placing your bladed hand against his neck.

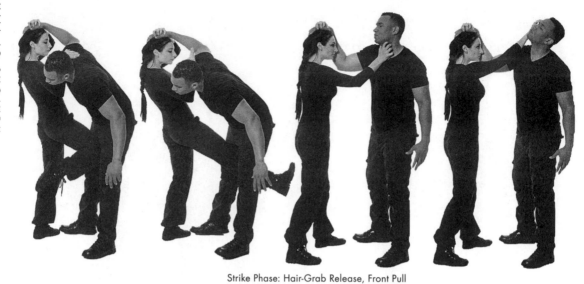

Strike Phase: Hair-Grab Release, Front Pull

Strike: Perform at least three Combative Knees to weaken his structure and grip.

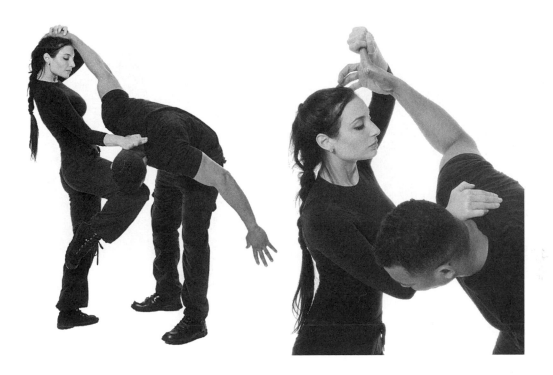

Survive: Peel the fingers from your hair. If he has a high tolerance for pain, be prepared to do an Eye Gouge or any combative that will bring him down.

Ground-Range Choking

Stop: Perform a Brace and a Single Hand Pluck with a simultaneous Palm Strike. (To brace, drive your shin across his hips and place the heel of your foot on his hipbone as a control and reference point.) By bracing your legs, you create a gate across the attacker's hips, and you'll be surprised how much power and control your legs can generate. Stop or release the choke by plucking the hand toward the side of your heel reference point. Bring your other hand in between his arms and do a Palm Strike, targeting his face.

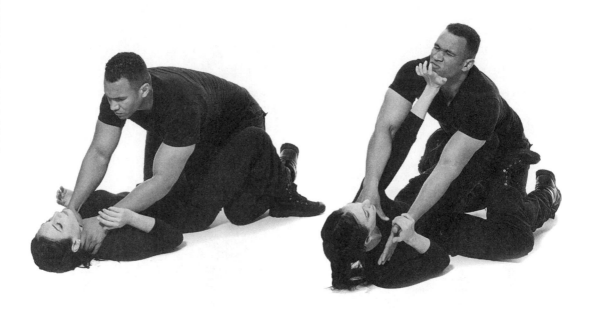

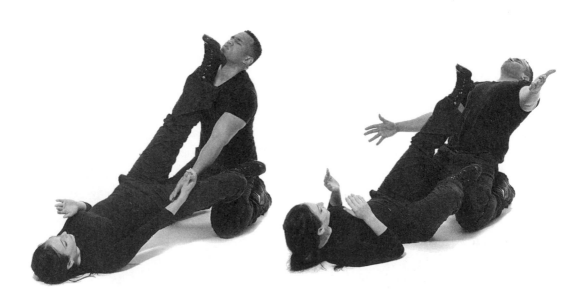

Secure: Keep hold of that plucked hand for temporary control. To maintain a temporary control over his grip, execute the Palm Strike just enough to create more space between his body and your brace leg—so that you can prepare to kick with the brace leg in the next phase.

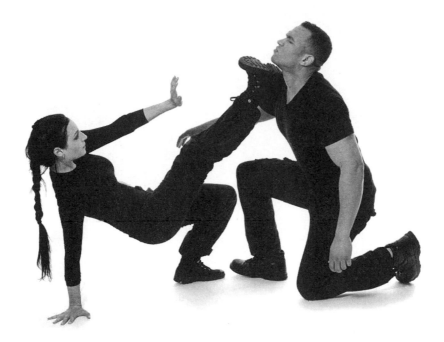

Strike: Push Kick the attacker in the face by driving your heel into his chin. This will send him backward. When you sit up, prepare to do another Push Kick in case he recovers quickly. Remember, you are training to adapt to the unknown.

Survive: Once you have confirmed that he is down, you have completed the steps necessary to get up, but make sure you do so safely: Face the attacker, take a step backward, and prepare to do Defensive Push Kicks along the way until you reach full Survival Stance. Don't assume that once you attempt to get back on your feet, you won't face another attack. While it is very common for people to just stand up whatever way feels comfortable, make sure you practice how to get up safely by following these simple steps:

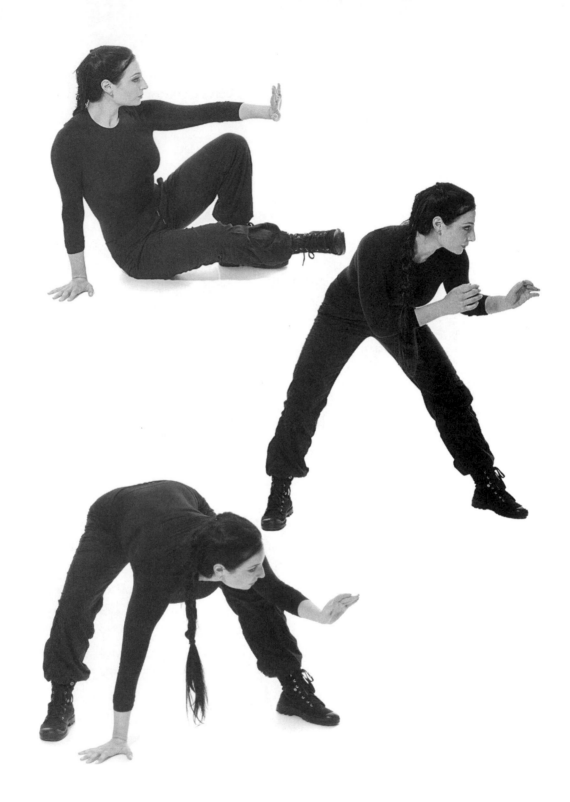

1 Place your rear-side hand on the ground.
2 Drive your kicking leg backward so that it is behind your supporting hand on the ground. It helps if you raise your hips.
3 Once your foot is flat on the ground, raise your chest to return to your full Survival Stance.

VISUALIZATION

Visualization is the bedrock of much of my self-defense training plan. As we continue to learn tactics and concepts, I want to make sure that you are able to experience your training in real-life scenarios. Remember that physical and mental freeze we talked about when you learned about the RACE Reaction Model? Well, in order to have the ability to overcome those freezes and build an authentic survival mindset, you will need to practice visualization; this will allow you to create fake "real experiences" for your mind to draw from when composing a defense against the threat or act of violence.

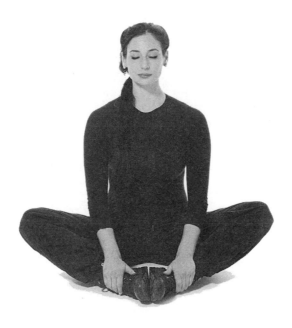

Visualizing has been my best secret weapon for all forms of success in my life. Starting with self-defense, I used visualization to retain the mechanics and movements of concepts while learning how to apply them in imagined locations, my "mental streets." Visualization also helped me retain my skill set when I was not able to train for months at a time. Then, when I started integrating combatives and a self-defense twist into my own personal workouts, I realized that as I was visualizing the combative component of each exercise, not only was I building my muscle memory, but I wasn't even aware of the pain or number of repetitions I had left in the set. Finally, my ability to visualize permeated every other aspect of my life and led me to visualize the life I wanted to have and the steps I needed to create and take to get there.

My ability to visualize has led to my finding happiness, purpose, and a new form of strength to apply to every aspect of my life. I have visualized the world that I wanted to live in, the moments that I would dedicate myself to living, and the possibility of getting everything I want out of life.

In practical terms, here's how to visualize:

Step 1: Find a quiet spot where nothing will distract you, and close your eyes. Picture yourself in a realistic setting—for example, the subway stop near your office, or the street outside your favorite cafe, or wherever. I recommend starting with selecting locations that you frequent and that are relevant to your life.

Step 2: As you are living in your imagined location, tune into all five of your senses: sight, hearing, touch, smell, and taste. Your surroundings will come to life as you begin to experience other elements such as temperature and other people around you. Notice small details such as the sound of birds (as an example).

Step 3: Create the threat. Select a suspicious person or imagine an attack that you would like to train, and go through your reaction. For example, picture a suspicious figure coming toward you. Immediately look at his hands—is he carrying any kind of weapon? Look at his face. Does he appear aggressive? Look around you. Are there any real exits that will provide an immediate and certain escape? If yes, run now. If no, formulate an action plan. Step into your Hidden Survival Stance and say "Okay." Then picture him striking you, and picture yourself using a combination of a block and combatives you've learned so far to disable him, take him down, and escape. Or simply visualize breaking the angle to gain a better position to scan your surroundings or advance with more combatives.

Step 4: Best-to-Worst Case. Experience your reactions to an attack in scenarios from the best case to the worst case. When I started doing this on my own, I began to see the value of going through some of my greatest fears and getting my mind conditioned to the reality of what could happen. I found this stage to have the most impact because I was able to practice the physical tactics with the strategics at the same time as I conditioned my survival mindset to extend beyond boundaries that would contribute to my freeze reactions.

Visualization will be a huge part of your training, so make sure you get comfortable with it. As you can see in the example above, you will be able to visualize your reaction in a way that will allow you to train your mind to adapt to the variables you could face on the street—which makes it realistic. Remember, your only objective is to survive at all costs; and when you start to visualize yourself completing combatives and defenses, you will begin to see a direct application to the life you know you can create. Surviving an attack is no different from getting through the next steps to reach your personal goal for what you want to achieve. I learned how to visualize the things that I wanted and the moments I wanted to experience, which helped me break down the steps I needed to take to get there.

Recap: How to Visualize

Drill Part 1: Create Your Surroundings: Spend two minutes "living" in a location in your mind by visualizing the elements and details. Start with locations you know and pay attention to the details. Focus on your senses to help you bring the location to life.

Drill Part 2: Tactics: Now that you are "living" in your visualized location, practice performing combatives and your defensive strategies as if you are facing
a real attack through the spectrum of best- to worst-case scenario.

Repetitions: I recommend repeating this full drill in five different imagined
locations.

HITTING YOUR TARGETS

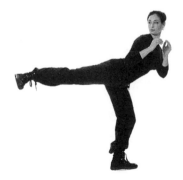

WEAPONS OF FITNESS

Now that you have seen the powerful weapon you can become, learned the stances, combatives, and defenses, and psyched yourself up, it's time to apply these to the *Weapons of Fitness* workouts. This chapter will take you through the some basic principles of the workouts, including the following:

1 *Weapons of Fitness* Warm-Up and Cooldown
2 Your Weapon of Strengthening
3 Your Weapon of Cardio
4 Your Weapon of Nutrition
5 Fitness Placement Test

WEAPONS OF FITNESS WARM-UP AND COOLDOWN

Warming up before a workout and completing a cooldown afterward are crucial to training safely and preventing injuries. Your warm-up will consist of light and easy movements to get your heart rate up and the blood flowing through your body before you complete a full body stretch. I recommend getting the heart rate up with a light jog or some skips on the spot.

Warm-Up Stretch: This should take about 10 minutes. I begin my warm-up stretch in a neutral stance and work from my neck all the way down to my ankles. Use my warm-up flow as a starting point, then add your favorite stretches into the mix.

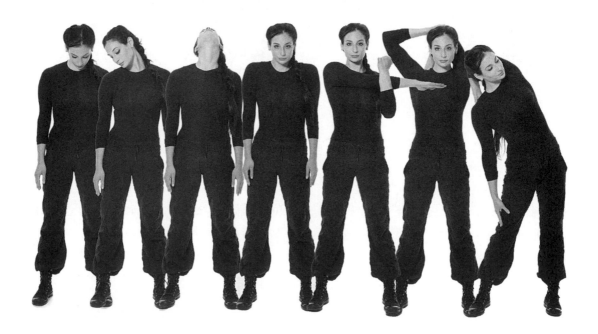

Make sure to do this warm-up on the right and left sides. Starting with your neck, circle your head first in one direction and then the other to start to loosen up your upper body. Transition down your body to your shoulders, raising and rotating them forward and backward. Next, bring your right arm across your body to further stretch your shoulder and keep it in place by hooking it in your left arm. Even though this is a common stretch, focus on the required hook position, as it is exactly the same hook needed for your Control Holds. Bring your left arm across your body and repeat the stretch. Then stretch out your triceps by bending your right arm and grabbing your elbow joint behind your head; then stretch your left tricep. Immediately transition into a side stretch by leaning your body to the right and then the left; you should feel the entire sides of your torso stretch and relax.

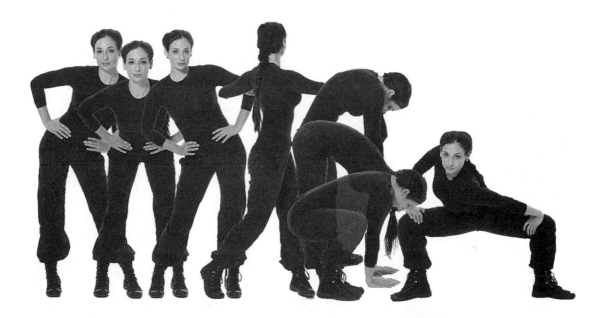

A Note About Stretching

WHEN YOU'RE DOING DYNAMIC STRETCHES (STRETCHES THAT REQUIRE YOU TO move while you do them), move at a regular and comfortable pace so that you can feel the muscles stretching and relaxing. When doing static stretches (those when the body is not moving), hold each one for 10 seconds and ease into it. If your muscles are tight, slowly get into the closest position possible and don't worry if you need to repeat the transition a couple of times. I would rather you be safe and increase your flexibility gradually than rush and get hurt.

As you work your way down your body, focus on loosening your hips by circling them to the right and the left. Complete at least 5 circles in each direction. Next, complete at least 5 torso twists by rotating your shoulders and pivoting on the ball of your foot (the same as you will need to do when striking!). Strive to face the rear wall as you relax and twist your torso. Then curl your body down until your hands touch the ground. As soon as your hands touch the ground, bend your knees to lower your hips, then reverse the process so that your hips lead your return and your head is the last part of your body to return to the upright position. Complete this transition at least 5 times. For the next stretch, work your way into an open squat—or a second-position plié, as I was taught in classical ballet—which will loosen up your hips. To get the full stretch, place both hands on your knees and let your hips sink down. Once you sink your hips, rotate each shoulder inward to keep your upper body stretching.

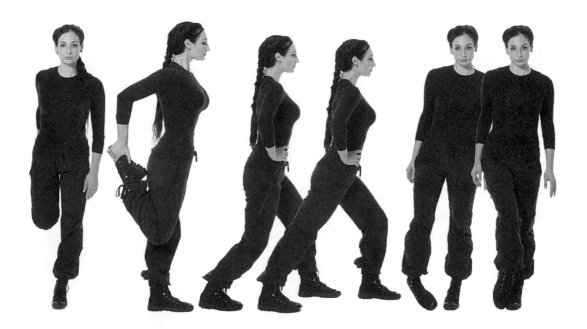

Next, stand up and grab your right heel to initiate a quad stretch. Make sure that you fight to keep both knees together as you simultaneously endeavor to keep your hips tucked in. Once you have completed your quad stretch on both sides, transition into your calf stretch. Stretch both the upper and lower calf by standing in a lunge position with your back knee straight and then bending it once you work your way down your calf muscle. Complete at least 2 full transitions of this stretch between the upper and lower calf muscle. Switch the position of your legs and repeat. Finally, make sure to warm up your ankles by completing basic circles in both directions. I also recommend circling your wrists during your warm-up, especially as the Soteria Method works your hands in a variety of moves.

Combative Warm-Up: Once you've stretched and limbered up, pick your favorite combative and do it 10 times in a row on one side, then do 10 jumping jacks. Now do the same combative on the other side (using your other hand, with your other foot forward), followed by another 10 jumping jacks. That counts as 1 set. Now pick another combative and repeat the sequence, bringing your total up to 2 sets. Complete 10 different combatives followed by 10 jumping jacks to finish up your warm-up, getting your blood moving and your heart rate up. With every set, gradually increase your speed by 10 percent until you reach 80 percent of your full speed or the 10 minutes is up.

YOUR WEAPON OF STRENGTHENING

In the next few chapters, as you get into the nitty-gritty of the workouts, I'll have you doing cardio regularly. Why and how?

Objective: Your objective is to create a lean and feminine figure that can ably defend itself against violence. This means that you need to focus on lengthening and contracting your targeted muscles to build long and lean muscle. The benefits of building long and lean muscle include improved power, improved muscle tone, boosted metabolism, reduced body fat, and increased prevention against diseases such as diabetes, arthritis, and heart disease.

Primary Targets: Core, glutes, arms. When I focused on these three primary areas, I was blown away by how quickly I was able to sculpt and shape my ultimate feminine figure. Every single *Weapons of Fitness* workout will cover all these areas as you get your heart rate up and burn fat.

My workouts are purely functional. You will use your whole body as a unit to complete every exercise. Our bodies are designed to move as a unit, and this will allow us to recruit even some of the most difficult muscles to target. This is also how we must condition our bodies for survival.

Weekly Commitment: You will commit to doing three to five workouts a week, depending on your personal goals. You will need to schedule these workouts in advance, which will help you commit to them, by filling in the charts I've provided in the following chapters. I recommend completing three or four workouts per week for general fitness and four or five workouts per week if you are an athlete or if your objective is to increase your endurance level.

REGARDLESS OF YOUR level, each workout will take around 30 minutes and will have the same structure, though this does not take into account the warm-up or the cooldown, which I leave to you to tailor to your own body.

Improvised Weapon Bonus Workout

AN IMPROVISED WEAPON IS ANY OBJECT THAT YOU CAN TURN INTO A WEAPON for self-protection. I will show you how to incorporate any object into your self-defense and fitness training, whether you are using it to distract or to actually disable an attacker. I won't say any more right now, but we are going to have fun in Chapter 12!

YOUR WEAPON OF CARDIO

Cardio plays an important role in overall health by exercising the heart muscle, helping you sustain prolonged levels of activity and burning fat. Many different cardio exercises can help you achieve your personal goals. Through my journey of sculpting and fighting, I was able to transition into doing cardio by completing rounds of continuous combatives, and I've never looked back.

Continuous combatives are the most effective and efficient way to progress through a series of movements. As you can see in the images opposite, you blend the return of one combative into the outgoing movement of another, as you would if you were using these moves in a real-life situation.

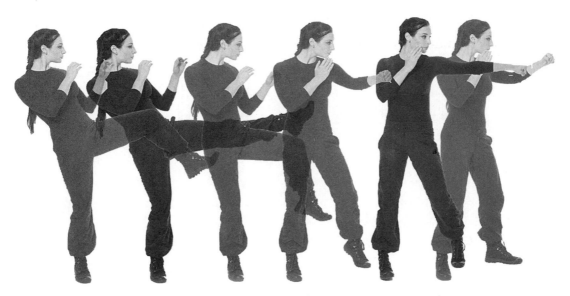

Continuous Combatives

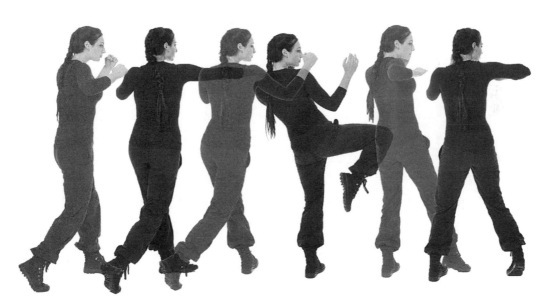

Continuous Combatives

Tips for Doing Continuous Combatives

BY BLENDING ONE COMBATIVE INTO THE NEXT, YOU ELIMINATE ANY PAUSE OR hesitation that could leave you open or vulnerable to a counter by the attacker. Not only do you complete more combatives in less time, but you also reduce the moments of stalling or freezing that an attacker can use against you. Take note that you want to initiate with the closer leg, and continue to use the next available near combative. When you go freestyle and do any combination that you want, try to complete no more than three upper-body combatives in a row or three lower-body combatives in a row; vary your target and striking surface area.

Whether you use continuous combatives in your offensive or defensive combative tactics, or in your strategies and techniques, you will effectively eliminate any telegraphing of your next move and make it extremely difficult for your aggressor to assess what you are doing. This will also help to prevent an attacker from formulating a reaction, as you disrupt his thought process over and over again.

Fitness Benefits: You are not only burning calories but also continuously elongating and contracting your muscles in a variety of ways, as opposed to doing a standard repetitive movement such as running. This will result in a greater range of contraction and recruit muscles that aren't traditionally utilized—allowing for a full-body transformation and workout. So whether you are performing continuous strikes, transitioning through phases of a defense, or getting the best cardio workout, this concept will serve to improve your coordination, agility, and timing for both self-defense and fitness.

This form of cardio can be adapted to meet your specific training objectives. If you want to target fat via a long, low-intensity aerobic session, you can perform the combatives within 60 to 75 percent of your maximum heart rate. If you want more intensity, do them faster. But always, always maintain perfect form and technique. In your training, technique is far more important than speed.

YOUR WEAPON OF CARDIO

With the right training drills, you will be able to execute continuous combatives without thinking. It will come naturally as you begin to move continuously, never stopping, but still being effective—every single second. Here are some great basic combination drills to get you started. They are simple and will allow you to gain the correct coordination and timing between your upper-body motions and lower-body motions.

DRILL 1

✳ Lower-Body Basic Footwork with Upper-Body Combatives

Description • This is a timing drill specifically designed to introduce the coordination needed to engage in upper-body combatives while traveling (moving) and using the lower body.

How-To • Get in Survival Stance. Maintain perfect form in your Survival Stance as you travel forward and backward, left and right. With each step you take, do a leading Straight Palm Strike with the near-side step and a Rear Palm Strike with the rear-side step. Please note that you can substitute the Palm Strike with any other upper-body combative that you want to focus on.

DRILL 2

✳ Snap Kick, Near Palm Strike, Rear Palm Strike, Snap Kick

Description • This drill requires you to perform the combination over and over from alternate sides and stances—an important thing to practice.

How-To • Engage in this combination traveling forward in a continuous manner so that one combative leads into the next. If you are a beginner, do this no faster than 20 percent of real time at first to ensure that your technique and form are correct and that you are applying the continuous factor of this concept correctly. Once you feel comfortable, increase the speed but maintain the proper technical execution of each strike.

As you become more advanced with this drill, perform this same combination traveling backward, and then try to perform the same combination on the spot. Both of these advanced versions will help bring you to the next level of controlling your positions—and tactically controlling your distance, angles, and overall defensive ranges.

DRILL 3

❋ Defensive Knee, Horizontal Elbow, Sky Elbow

Description • This combination solely engages close-range power combatives. Start off slow, increase your speed, and then attempt to engage in the combative traveling backward and also on the spot. This is your "shadow boxing" drill, designed to allow you to engage in random combatives following the principles of continuous combatives. You can bring in the mental challenge of imagining someone in front of you and countering his actions. This is also a great way to warm up before a training session and one of the best ways to burn calories and boost your metabolism.

ADVANCED DRILLS

❋ Random Continuous Combatives, Random Continuous Combatives with Travel, Dry Defenses (adding in your defenses too!)

Drill Recommendations • Put on your favorite playlist and work the shadow boxing in intervals using variables such as speed or limiting yourself to close-range or long-range combatives. You can also bring in the variable of distance and how much distance you incorporate into various combinations. Also change your angles so you work off multiple reference points.

How to Add Aerobic Cardio to Your Workouts

IN SIMPLE TERMS, "AEROBIC" EXERCISE MEANS YOU'RE DOING CONTINUOUS movement in which your muscles require oxygen for fuel. Below are the key elements of the continuous combative cardio that I want you doing:

Intensity: The intensity is outlined as between 60 to 75 percent of your maximum heart rate. To find your maximum heart rate, simply subtract your age from 220. So, use the formula (220 − your age) × .75 to find out what is 75 percent of your max heart rate. Don't exceed this number.

Time of Day: I recommend doing cardio first thing in the morning or right after a *Weapons of Fitness* workout, but ultimately, I want you to get your cardio sessions in when it is good for you and your lifestyle.

Duration: I recommend 20 to 40 minutes of cardio, either doing 30 to 40 minutes of cardio in the morning, or adding 20 to 30 minutes of cardio after you have completed a *Weapons of Fitness* workout. Please note that the *Weapons of Fitness* workouts are full-body-conditioning workouts that incorporate both strengthening and cardio, as you will elevate your heart rate while targeting core muscle groups.

Forms of Cardio: My favorite cardio routine is doing interval continuous combatives. I understand that some of you will have your own favorite method and some of you will require certain forms of cardio for athletic ability or injury recovery. For this reason, I want you to make the cardio work for you and transition over to continuous combatives when you feel ready. Feel free to build the duration of the continuous combative routine gradually, and to complete the remainder of your cardio session with your own form, such as running, swimming, biking, power walking, or using standard gym machines like the elliptical. Jumping rope is also a great cardio activity, and one of my favorites.

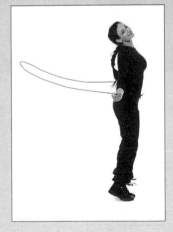

Interval Continuous Combatives

INTEGRATING HIGH-INTENSITY INTERVAL TRAINING IN YOUR ROUTINE WORKS your anaerobic energy system (as opposed to your aerobic energy system). This structure helps you to improve your overall endurance and your ability to go from 0 to 100 percent in an instant, which is something you'll need to do if you are suddenly attacked on the street.

For those at the beginner and intermediate levels, complete 10 to 20 rounds of 20 seconds of continuous combatives at high speed (90 percent of maximum heart rate), and 10 to 20 rounds of 40 seconds at resting speed (50 percent); the whole practice should take between 10 and 20 minutes, depending on how many rounds you do.

For those at the advanced and advanced plus levels, complete 20 seconds at high speed (90 percent), followed by 20 seconds at resting speed (50 percent). Repeat this combination for 10 to 20 rounds.

Interval training will condition your body to react more efficiently during an adrenaline surge. This is similar to the physical demands that will be placed on you when your heart rate and adrenaline levels are high.

YOUR WEAPON OF NUTRITION

I endorse a lifestyle of nutrition, not a diet. I initially designed the *Weapons of Fitness* nutritional guidelines for myself. They are full of positive steps to take and habits to form to finally overcome all the negative preconceptions, beliefs, and pressures associated with diets. I've spent a lot of time throughout my life feeling bad about my body because of some perceived norm or definition of beauty—and those are days of my life that I won't get back. When I finally redefined self-defense for myself, my approach to dieting changed as well. I became focused on what I wanted to create in my life and saw my body as the vehicle to turn my dreams into reality. When that happened, food became just the fuel that I needed to burn to keep my body running. I was able to make the shift from living to eat to eating to live.

I know it is easier said than done, but these guidelines not only made me feel better about myself and my body but also led me to lose all of the weight that I wanted. These guidelines ask you to adopt new long-term habits with a sustainable new mindset. If you are anything like I used to be (signing on for restrictive diets and then losing control at mealtime and descending into a guilt-failure spiral), then it is time to take a deep breath and relax. These nutritional guidelines will set you free.

You can tackle one habit at a time, or change everything according to the complete guidelines. Regardless, you will still be selecting foods that you like and making changes that fit with your lifestyle—and yes, we will celebrate cheats together!

Nutritional Guidelines

Habit 1: Limit Your Consumption of These Five Bad Guys

1 Fried foods: This is obvious. If it's fried, don't touch it. There are many better alternatives.

2 Processed sugar: Try to cut out as much as you can from your diet. Processed-sugar-laden foods to avoid include candies, baked goods, cereals, and soda and fruit-flavored drinks.

3 High-sodium foods: Avoid processed and prepackaged foods, which often have a very high sodium content.

4 Alcohol: Drink alcohol only in moderate amounts, so you can avoid the extra calories in these beverages.

5 Red meats and processed meats: Limiting your consumption of red and processed meats is a good way to avoid the fats and additives found in these products.

Habit 2: Eat Smaller Meals Every Three to Four Hours. For me, this means four to six times a day. This will help you avoid going into "starvation mode" and holding on to every last calorie for dear life—or succumbing to hunger and going on a junk-food binge mid-afternoon because the gap between lunch and dinner is too long.

Habit 3: Hydrate! Drink 1.5 to 3 liters (approximately 50 to 100 ounces) of water per day. A great way to start is by drinking a large glass of water before each meal. The more water you drink, the more your body flushes out toxins, helping you to maintain the proper amount of water in your cells and optimizing the functionality of your organ systems.

Habit 4: Avoid Carbs Before Bed. Don't eat carbohydrates three hours before bedtime. This is a great habit to get into, as many of us tend to snack in the evenings (especially when in front of the computer or television). And often these "snacks" end up with our consuming many more calories than expected—as in "I can't believe I ate the whole bag of chips!"

Habit 5: Eat Whole Foods Only! This is bringing your diet back to basics—food groups found in nature and prepared in the least invasive way to maintain nutritional integrity. This will bring you back to appreciating naturally sweet foods too.

Habit 6: Exercise Portion Control. Again, moderation is key here. For example, a large salad two or three times a day is proportional. However, eating buckets and buckets of salad is not necessary to maintain good health.

Habit 7: Plan Ahead. Try to eliminate the chance that you won't have ingredients to prepare meals at home—for the day or for the workweek ahead—so that you aren't forced to buy junk food. Find the best day of the week (I like Sundays) to prepare some meals for the week ahead, such as soups, stews, and healthy baked goods.

Habit 8: Give Yourself a Fighting Chance. Stock your fridge and pantry with healthy snacks. It is just as easy to reach for a piece of fruit as it is to grab a package of cookies!

Habit 9: Start Your Day with a Good Meal. Breakfast is the most important meal of the day. A nutritionally rich meal in the morning will set you up for success, giving you increased energy, greater concentration, and the ability to ignore calorie heavy but nutritionally empty food choices from food carts, vending machines, and the counter of your favorite coffee shop.

Habit 10: Pay Attention to Your Food Habits. If you take the time to examine your food choices and eating habits, you will recognize areas that you would like to change. You do not need to change everything at once, but do make an ongoing effort to change each unwanted habit so that the result is a diet rich in nutritional foods that are eaten in moderation and overall better health.

Habit 11: Substitute Healthier Options. When it comes to food options, choose those with fewer calories and fewer carbohydrates. For example, drinking a hot cup of herbal tea (such as green tea) is a much better alternative than having a mega-size cappuccino with extra whipped topping and chocolate shavings. Of course, there will always be times when you crave a high-calorie beverage—so plan accordingly and make sure your intake for the day can accommodate these extra calories.

Habit 12: Make Mealtime an Occasion. Sit down and have your meal at the table—not in front of the television, at the computer, or while driving or reading. Setting aside a time to simply sit at the table and be present during the meal is a great opportunity to reflect on your day and/or spend quality time with family and friends.

Habit 13: Stop Eating When You Are Done. Be mindful of the fact that it takes about 20 minutes for your body to register the amount of food you have consumed. Many people have attributed weight loss to eating more slowly, which has led to lower caloric intakes at each sitting. Focus on enjoying your food and don't worry about cleaning your plate (sorry, Mom!). Remember, it is about quality, not quantity, and your body will thank you for it!

Habit 14: Sleep! The amount of sleep you get can have a direct impact on how you approach eating. If you are tired or grumpy, you will often find yourself reaching for something to munch on—if only to keep yourself awake with the chewing noises!

Habit 15: Hang Out with These Food-Group Friends. Here are the food groups you should be spending the most mealtime with: whole grains, proteins (fish, beans, nuts, and poultry), healthy fats (nuts, plant oils, and fish). Limit foods high in saturated fats (red meats, whole-milk products) and avoid those with trans fats (shortenings, baked goods, processed foods).

Habit 16: Let Fruits and Vegetables Rule! The more colorful your fruit and vegetable choices, the greater their nutritional benefits to your diet. Go ahead and try varieties you may not be familiar with—that odd-looking vegetable with the weird leaves could become your new favorite!

Habit 17: Get Enough Calcium. Calcium is an important part of your diet, but it isn't necessarily best gotten from milk products. Dark green leafy vegetables also have high levels of calcium.

Habit 18: Notice the "Why" of Your Eating. Pay attention to those times when you eat while distracted. Are you eating when you are upset? When you are worried? When you are angry? When you are down? Look for clues to your emotional eating and make a conscious effort to break this bond; you *can* unlearn this connection and greatly reduce your calorie intake. There are other solutions for dealing with stress, and one of the best is exercise!

Habit 19: Exercise Away Your Route to the Fridge. Find a way to substitute a physical activity for a trip to the fridge or the cupboard. This can mean simply getting outside and walking around the block. Plan to make fitness a greater part of your life and you will find that eating for the sake of eating becomes less and less compelling.

Habit 20: You Can (and Should) Treat Yourself on Occasion. When you're at a party and want to enjoy a piece of cake, have it! Just be aware that you should not volunteer to take home the remaining slab of cake if you cannot ignore it in your fridge. By consciously allowing yourself the occasional treat, you actually reinforce your ability to eat in moderation and with purpose—to maintain your health.

FITNESS PLACEMENT TEST

Before you jump into Week 1 of the workouts, you need to determine your best starting point. The *Weapons of Fitness* workouts are broken down into beginner, intermediate, advanced, and advanced plus levels. You can start at any level (though I hope you'll begin with the one determined from the results of your Fitness Placement Test), and move to a more or less advanced level if you need to adjust once you're already under way.

The fitness test is simple: Perform as many repetitions of each the following six basic fitness exercises as you can in 1 minute. Use the chart on the next page to record your results. Remember, you are supposed to complete as many as you can in 1 minute. Don't fake it and go for 90 seconds to impress me! You'll only be cheating yourself.

Calculate your results: Look at columns 2, 3, 4, and 5 of the Fitness Test Results table below and give yourself a score for each activity: 1 for beginner, 2 for intermediate, 3 for advanced, and 4 for advanced plus. Once you've recorded your results, calculate your average: Add up all your results and divide that number by 6 and round down to see where you place on the rating scale. Start your workouts in the appropriate bracket.

In columns 6 and 7 of the chart that follows, I've filled out some sample results. Fill in your own results in the blank chart below.

FITNESS TEST RESULTS						
Task: For all of the below, perform as many as you can in a row without pausing for a break.						
Test	Beginner (B)	Intermediate (I)	Advanced (A)	Advanced+ (A+)	Your Results (Please list B, I, A, or A+)	Score (1–4) See values below
Squats	< 15	16–30	31–45	> 45		
Lunges	< 15	16–30	31–45	> 45		
Push-Ups	< 10	11–25	26 to 45	> 45		
Sit-ups	< 10	11–30	31–60	> 60		
Planks	< 20 sec.	20 sec.–1 min.	> 1 min.	> 2 min.		
Burpees	1 to 3	4 to 10	11 to 20	> 20		
Congrats! Your starting point is:						
Remember: Beginner = 1 Intermediate = 2 Advanced = 3 Advanced+ = 4						

FITNESS TEST RESULTS	
Task: For all of the below, perform as many as you can in a row without pausing for a break.	
Your Results (Please list B, I, A, or A+)	Score (1–4) See values below
Congrats! Your starting point is:	
Remember: Beginner = 1 Intermediate = 2 Advanced = 3 Advanced+ = 4	

EXERCISE 1

 Squat

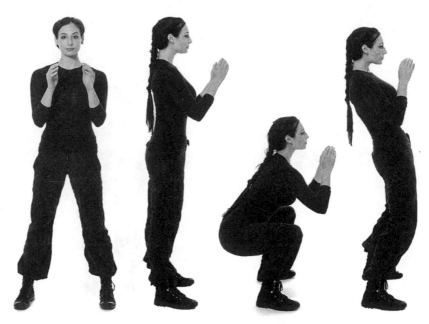

Starting Position • Off-Guard Stance

Movement • Drive your hips back and down until your thighs (or femurs) are parallel to the ground. Keep your head up and your chest raised as you lower your hips. Make sure that your knees don't go farther forward than your toes, which will protect your knees. Engage your glutes and visualize your glutes lifting you as you stand back up. As you return to starting position, complete your full range of motion by tucking in the pelvis; this will help you make the most of every repetition.

Tip • The closer together your feet are, the more you run the risk of placing pressure on your knees, so make sure that you start in a neutral stance with your feet slighter wider than shoulder-width apart; you can even flare your feet outward slightly to help with balance and alignment.

EXERCISE 2

✸ Lunge

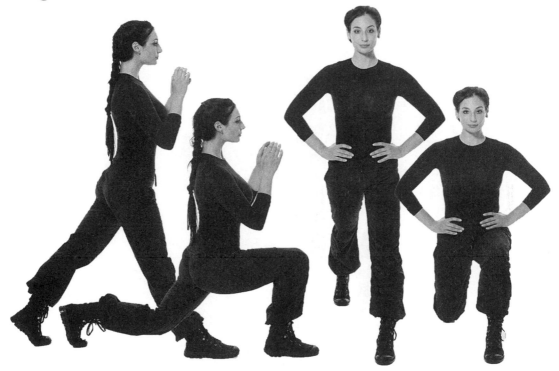

Starting Position • From a standing position with both feet together, establish your starting position by taking a deep step back with one leg directly behind you (make sure you have significant distance between each leg).

Movement • Drop your hips down so that your front thigh is parallel to the ground. Keep your chest raised and make sure that your front knee does not move beyond your front foot. As you raise your hips to return to the starting position, engage your glutes.

✹ Push-Up

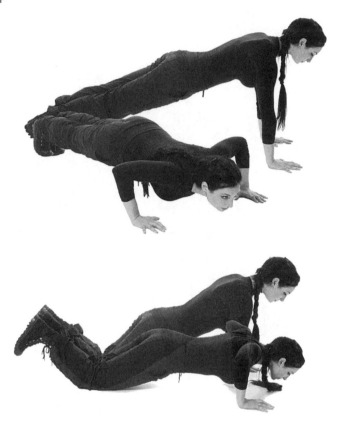

Starting Position • Plank position. To target the chest, shoulders, and triceps, you want to place your hands right below or slightly lower than the plane of your shoulders. Make sure that you maintain a straight line running from your head through your neck and down to your spine so that your body is flat and your hips are not dipping or raised too much.

Movement • Drop your chest about 1 to 2 inches above the ground. As you achieve your full range of motion, maintain the straight line of your torso to help target and engage the core as well. To complete the movement, use your arms to push your chest back up to the starting position.

Tip • If it is difficult to complete 1 repetition on your toes, complete the push-up on your knees, following the same guidelines outlined above.

EXERCISE 4

❊ Sit-Up

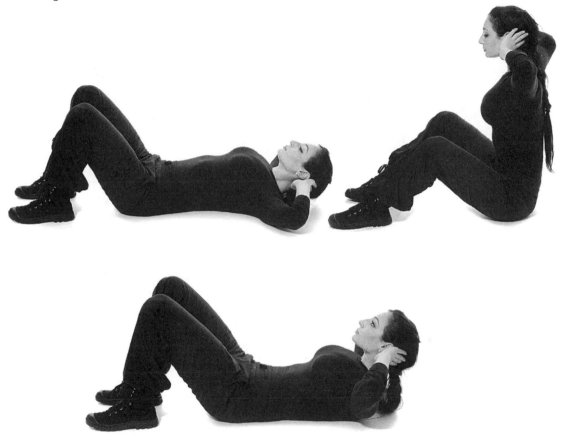

Starting Position • Lying on your back with your knees bent and your feet on the ground, with both hands behind your head and your elbows flared out to open up your chest.

Movement • Drive your upper body with your chest toward the ceiling and eventually to meet the tops of your knees/thighs. Return to the ground to complete 1 repetition.

EXERCISE 5

✸ Plank

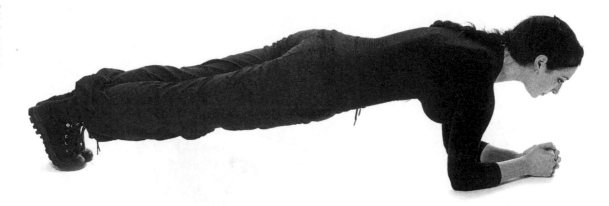

Starting Position • Instead of supporting your body with your hands, as you did for the push-up, support your body with your forearms. Keep a straight line from your head through your neck and torso and all the way down to your toes.

Movement • There is no movement. This is a static hold, so fight not to let your hips drop down or raise too high. Hold the position as long as you can.

EXERCISE 6

✸ Burpee

Starting Position • Survival Stance (make sure there's plenty of space behind you)

Movement • From Survival Stance, drop down in a tucked position, place your hands by your front feet, and jump both legs back behind you into a sprawl. Then jump both legs back up, into your Survival Stance.

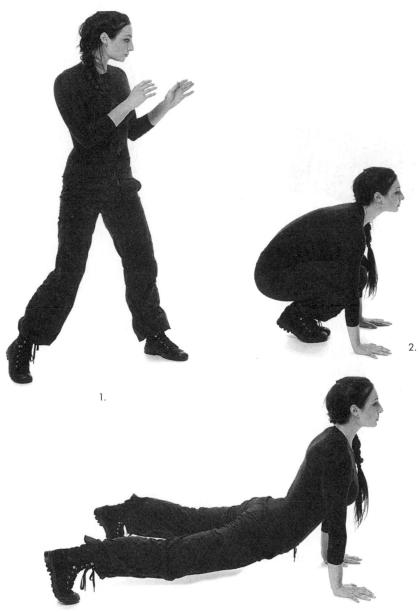

1.

2.

3.

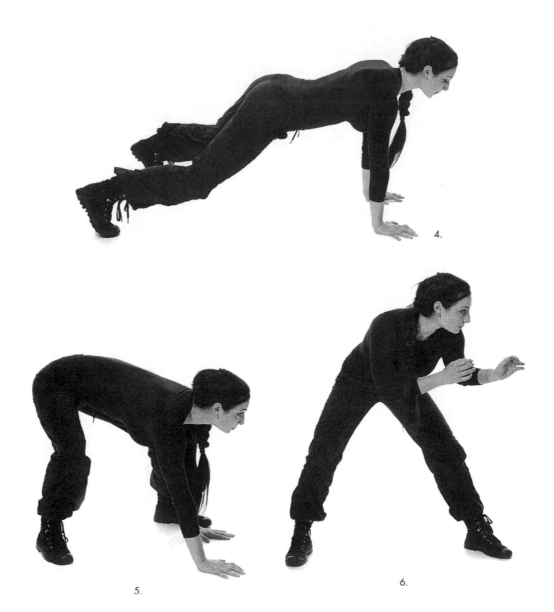

4.

5.

6.

SCHEDULING YOUR SUCCESS

I believe that success is something you prepare for by not leaving anything to chance. Schedule your workouts in advance, which is the best way to arm yourself to overcome any sudden weakness, wrong frame of mind, or tempting excuse that may arise. I have provided a sample workout schedule that I drew up for myself. In each of the next three chapters, I include blank charts so that you can fill out your workout schedule. Keep this book with you, and when you feel weak, take a look at the commitment you made—no excuses!

For the first week, you will complete three *Weapons of Fitness* workouts and one to three cardio combative sessions. Your cardio sessions should be based on the principles you learned in this chapter's "Weapon of Cardio" section, but feel free to personalize them if you like. After the first week, you can tweak the number of sessions depending on your training objectives and fitness level. I personally like to do cardio Monday, Wednesday, and Friday, first thing in the morning, on an empty stomach, for 30 to 40 minutes—and to complete my *Weapons of Fitness* workouts on Tuesday, Thursday, and Saturday afternoons/evenings.

SCHEDULE TRACKER							
Day of Week	Day 1	Day 2	Day 3	Day 4	Day 5	Day 6	Day 7
Weapons of Fitness							
Cardio Combatives							
Soteria Pyramid Minutes							
Visualization Minutes							
Nutrition							
Inner Soteria							

Use this chart to schedule your weekly workouts and training time, in additional to monitoring and tracking your achievements.

✳ Reading the Chart

Weapons of Fitness Workout • This is your primary workout routine, so make sure to schedule at least three workouts per week. I don't recommend exceeding five workouts a week—remember, your body needs time to rest and recover.

Cardio Combatives • Schedule at least two additional cardio sessions each week.

Soteria Method Survival Pyramid Minutes • Schedule at least 10 minutes dedicated to visualizing your combatives and self-defense reactions and to breaking down boundaries for your survival mindset to grow.

Visualization Minutes • After you complete reading and practicing a self-defense tactic or concept in this book, spend time visualizing yourself performing the concept in your mind.

Nutrition • At the end of each day of healthy, purposeful eating, write down "Clean" after you have taken your last bite at dinner. This will help reinforce that you are in control and have followed through on your word.

Inner Soteria • Dedicate at least 10 minutes in the morning to visualizing your success, both in self-defense and in life. Whether you choose to meditate or to simply relax for 10 minutes before work, use this time to reflect on what you want to create, visualize yourself creating it, and assign yourself at least one task to complete that day that will help you achieve it. Spend this time preparing your reaction to any difficult situation. This is where you will apply all the *Weapons of Fitness* concepts to your everyday life, knock out fear, and protect your outlook on who you are and what you have to offer.

WEEKS 1 AND 2 WORKOUTS

Welcome to your first two weeks of *Weapons of Fitness* training. As promised, here are your *Weapons of Fitness* schedules to fill in. I have also included the *Weapons of Fitness* workout structure at the beginning of each workout chapter to remind you of the order. The workouts will last for two weeks, and then you'll move on to the next chapter and learn a whole new routine to challenge your body for greater results.

Before you see the workout breakdown, I want you to fill out your first-week success tracker, which is the chart for you to schedule your workouts. After you've completed the first week, come back and fill in your second-week workout schedule (and feel free to try a more advanced exercise level).

SCHEDULE TRACKER							
Day of Week	Day 1	Day 2	Day 3	Day 4	Day 5	Day 6	Day 7
Weapons of Fitness							
Cardio Combatives							
Soteria Pyramid Minutes							
Visualization Minutes							
Nutrition							
Inner Soteria							

SCHEDULE TRACKER							
Day of Week	Day 1	Day 2	Day 3	Day 4	Day 5	Day 6	Day 7
Weapons of Fitness							
Cardio Combatives							
Soteria Pyramid Minutes							
Visualization Minutes							
Nutrition							
Inner Soteria							

WEAPONS OF FITNESS WEEKS 1 AND 2						
Exercise	Beginner	Intermediate	Advanced	Advanced +	Burnouts	Sets/Reps
Warm-Up						
Squat Blocks	12 Squats | 12 Blocks	12 Squats | 12 Blocks and Counters	12–15 Squat: Squat Blocks and Counters	12–15 Vertical Squat Blocks and Counters	30–60 seconds of alternating combatives OR Jumping Jacks OR Skips	3 Sets
Side Lunge Kicks	12 Side Lunges | 12 Side Kicks	12 Side Lunges | 12 Side Kicks	12 Side Lunges and Side Kicks	15 Side Lunges and Side Kicks		
Push-Up Elbows	8 Push-Up Elbows from knees	12 Push-Up Elbows from knees	8 Push-Up Elbows from feet	12 Push-Up Elbows from feet		
Self-Defense Burpees	8 Burpees into Survival Stance	12 Burpees into Survival Stance with Palm Strikes	12 Burpees into Survival Stance. with Kick, Palm Strike, Elbow	15 Burpees into Survival Stance, any combatives		
Heel Dips	10 Heel Dips per leg	12 Heel Dips per leg	10 Single Heel Dips into Raised Push Kick	15 Single Heel Dips into Raised Push Kick		
Cooldown and Stretch						

WEAPONS OF FITNESS WORKOUT BREAKDOWN

Here's how the *Weapons of Fitness* workouts are going to play out. Take a look at the charts on page 162 for Weeks 1 and 2 to see what each exercise entails and what makes up a repetition. More specific information for the beginner, intermediate, advanced, and advanced plus levels follows.

Warm-Up: • Warm up with dynamic stretches and combatives according to the instructions on pages 136–139.

Exercises • Do 3 sets of repetitions or timed durations for each exercise, making sure each set is followed by 1 minute of burnouts.

Cooldown • Take an easy walk and do some stretching.

Burnouts • As the name implies, you will burn out your body by performing continuous combatives as fast as you can. However, I have one rule: You must go only as fast as your technique lets you. Do not compromise technique for speed. Burnouts boost your heart rate and conditioning for self-defense. The more familiar and comfortable you get with the combatives, the faster you'll be able to do them in burnouts—and the faster you'll be able to do them in real life, if you ever need to use them. I also recommend challenging yourself by purchasing 1-pound weights and holding one weight in each hand during your burnout rounds to add more resistance.

EXERCISE 1

✻ Squat Blocks

Primary Fitness Targets • Glutes, core

Primary Self-Defense Target • Improves blocking reflexes

Starting Position • Off-Guard Stance

Movement • Full Squat | Block and Counter

Movement 1: Complete a full Squat (reference the Fitness Placement Test in Chapter 8 if needed), and as you return to starting position, tuck your pelvis for the full range of motion. Those who are advanced plus should add 1 jump in between 2 Squats to make it vertical.

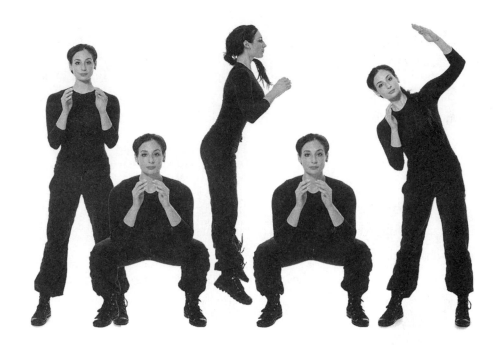

Movement 2: From your pelvis tuck, immediately go into a Block (beginner) or a Block and Counter (all other levels). Reference the "Blocking" section, in Chapter 7, to make sure your form is correct. This is a great opportunity to improve your blocking reflexes.

Beginner • 12 Squats | 12 Blocks—Complete your sets of Squats and Blocks separately. Make sure that you are building correct form for the Squat and the correct muscle memory for the Blocks. Maintain the same amount of optimal space between your face and arm in every rep you complete—this Block could help save your life against an active attack.

Intermediate • 12 Squats | 12 Blocks and Counters—Complete your sets of Squats and Blocks separately, and add in a Counter Palm Strike on each Block.

Advanced • 12 to 15 Squat Blocks and Counters—Blend the return of the Squat into the blocking position. Work from the Off-Guard Position for this exercise, because it will train your reflexive blocks in case you ever find yourself caught unaware.

Advanced Plus • 12 to 15 Vertical Squat Blocks and Counters—Add a vertical jump between two Squats and one Block with a simultaneous Counter.

EXERCISE 2

✸ Side Lunge Kicks

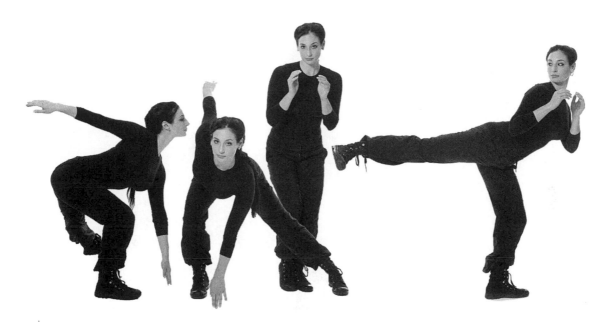

Primary Fitness Targets • Glutes, core

Primary Self-Defense Targets • Knee, groin

Starting Position • Standing with feet together

Movement • Side Lunge into a Side Kick

Movement 1: Take a deep side step into a Side Lunge. Make sure that you keep your hips back and that your knee does not pass your foot. Keep your chest up and return to the starting position.

Movement 2: As soon as you return from your Side Lunge, identify an imaginary target and execute the Side Kick. (Making eye contact with a specific target will help you work on your eye-body coordination.)

Beginner • 12 Side Lunges | 12 Side Kicks—Complete 12 Side Lunges in a row and then 12 Side Kicks in a row to isolate the movements.

Intermediate • 12 Side Lunges | 12 Side Kicks—Complete 12 Side Lunges in a row and then 12 Side Kicks in a row to isolate the movements.

Advanced • 12 Side Lunges and Side Kicks—Do 12 reps of a Side Lunge directly into a Side Kick.

Advanced Plus • 15 Side Lunges and Side Kicks—Do 15 reps of a Side Lunge directly into a Side Kick.

EXERCISE 3

✺ Push-Up Elbows

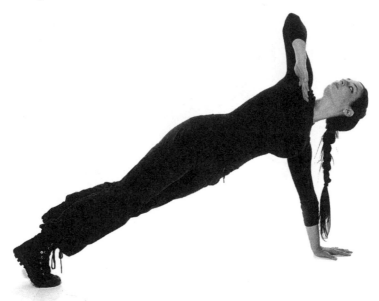

Primary Fitness Targets • Chest, arms

Primary Self-Defense Targets • Elbow to face

Starting Position • Plank

Movement • Push-Up into Swinging Rear Elbow

Movement 1: Push-Up (reference the Fitness Placement Test, in Chapter 8, if needed)

Movement 2: Swinging Rear Elbow. As soon as you return to a plank position from your Push-Up, swing one elbow up toward the ceiling as if you were going to make contact with someone directly on top of you. Meanwhile, rotate your core out to the same side and look up toward where your elbow is striking. This is a great drill to practice the twisting of the combative from an unconventional position, which helps reinforce the concept. I also recommend placing your focus on the three tips for forming a consistent elbow combative: Bladed Hand, Body Contact, and Extension (see Chapter 5).

Beginner • 8 Push-Up Elbows from knees

Intermediate • 12 Push-Up Elbows from knees

Advanced • 8 Push-Up Elbows from feet

Advanced Plus • 12 Push-Up Elbows from feet

EXERCISE 4

✸ Self-Defense Burpees

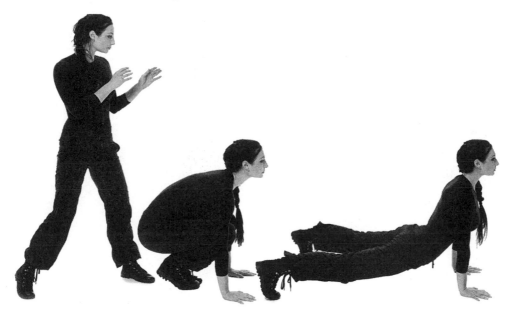

Primary Fitness Target • Glutes

Primary Self-Defense Target • Eyes

Starting Position • Survival Stance

Movement • Self-Defense Burpee | 2 Combatives

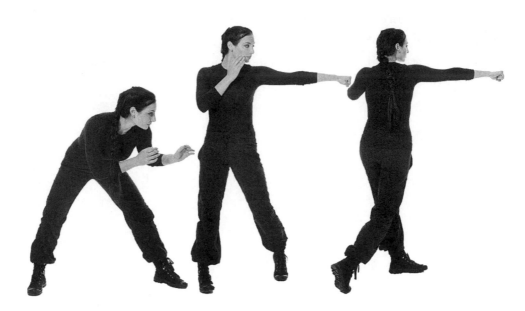

Movement 1: Complete a Burpee (reference the Fitness Placement Test, in Chapter 8, if needed). Make sure to return to Survival Stance after each Burpee.

Movement 2: Once you are in Survival Stance, immediately engage in combatives, such as the Palm Strike or the Hook Punch.

Beginner • 8 Burpees into Survival Stance

Intermediate • 12 Burpees into Survival Stance with Palm Strikes

Advanced • 12 Burpees into Survival Stance with Combative Combo: Kick, Palm Strike, Elbow

Advanced Plus • 15 Burpees into Survival Stance with any combatives you want to practice

EXERCISE 5

✹ Heel Dips

Primary Fitness Target • Core

Primary Self-Defense Target • Face

Starting Position • Back

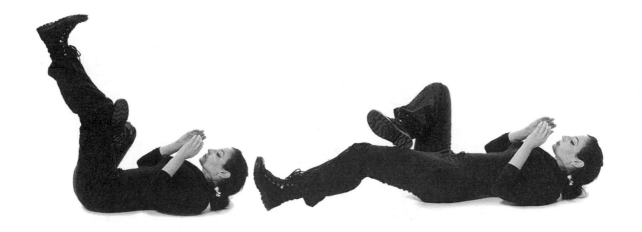

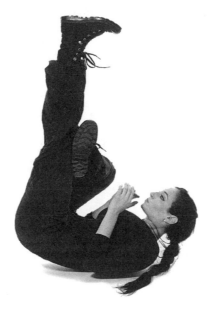

Movement • Heel Dip

Movement 1: Lie on your back with one leg pointed up in the air directly in front of you. Make sure your knee is slightly bent—similar to the angle you practiced when preparing to do a Push Kick. Make sure to keep the foot of your extended leg flexed, while you bring your other ankle across the thigh of your dipping leg. Your outer shin should be lying across the thigh of your dipping leg.

Maintain this position with your legs as you dip your heel to the ground for a second and raise it to return to the starting position. The trick here is not to let the leg rest on the ground, because then you let the core relax, and you want that full contraction so the core is engaged throughout the entire movement. As you complete the reps, I want you to focus on the elevated leg and how you will prep the Push Kick from both a standing and ground position.

Movement 2: For those at the advanced and advanced plus levels only, raise your hips and execute a Push Kick, as if to the face of an attacker who is advancing toward you when you are on your back.

Beginner • 10 Heel Dips per each leg

Intermediate • 12 Heel Dips per each leg

Advanced • Single Heel Dip into a single Push Kick per each leg. Repeat 10 times to complete the set.

Advanced Plus • 15 Heel Dips with a Push Kick per each leg

CARDIO COMBATIVE CHALLENGE

For Weeks 1 and 2, you will do a series of continuous combatives to your favorite music. Focus on performing the repetitions in each round without compromising your technique.

Complete the sequence below until you have reached your goal duration.

If you want to extend the cardio or do it for a specific duration, feel free to use this sequence and just simply repeat until you have reached your goal.

1 50 Alternating Upper Body Combatives | 30 Skips | 30 Jumping Jacks

2 20 Elbows per side | 30 Skips | 30 Jumping Jacks

3 20 Knees per side | 30 Skips | 30 Jumping Jacks

4 20 Push Kicks per side | 30 Skips | 30 Jumping Jacks

WEEKS 3 AND 4 WORKOUTS

C ongratulations on completing the first two weeks of the *Weapons of Fitness* workouts, and welcome to the next phase. Please fill in your training schedule below.

SCHEDULE TRACKER							
Day of Week	Day 1	Day 2	Day 3	Day 4	Day 5	Day 6	Day 7
Weapons of Fitness							
Cardio Combatives							
Soteria Pyramid Minutes							
Visualization Minutes							
Nutrition							
Inner Soteria							

SCHEDULE TRACKER							
Day of Week	Day 1	Day 2	Day 3	Day 4	Day 5	Day 6	Day 7
Weapons of Fitness							
Cardio Combatives							
Soteria Pyramid Minutes							
Visualization Minutes							
Nutrition							
Inner Soteria							

WEAPONS OF FITNESS WEEKS 3 AND 4						
Exercise	Beginner	Intermediate	Advanced	Advanced +	Burnouts	Sets/Reps
Warm-Up						
Squat Strikes	12 Squats with Palm Strikes	12 Squats, 2 Palm Strikes, 2 Elbow combatives	12 Squats with any 3 upper-body combatives	12–15 Vertical Squats, any 3 upper-body combatives	30–60 seconds of alternating combatives OR Jumping Jacks OR Skips	3 Sets
Forward Lunge Combatives	12 Lunges | 12 Push Kicks	12 Lunges | 12 Push Kicks and Elbows	12–15 Lunges, Push Kicks, and Elbows	12–15 Lunges into personal combative combination		
Tricep Kicking Get-Ups	8 Tricep Push Kicks	15 Tricep Push Kicks	8 Tricep Push Kicks with Get-Up	12 Tricep Push Kicks with Get-Up		
Speed Kicks	10–15 Speed Kicks	20–30 Speed Kicks	20 Speed Kicks at all angles	30–40 Speed Kicks at all angles		
Brace Crunches	12 Brace Crunches	30 Brace Crunches	45 Brace Crunches	60 Brace Crunches		
Cooldown and Stretch						

WEAPONS OF FITNESS WORKOUT BREAKDOWN

Warm-Up • Warm up with dynamic stretches and combatives according to the instructions on pages 138–141.

Exercises • Do 3 sets of repetitions or timed durations for each exercise, making sure each set is followed by 1 minute of burnouts.

Cooldown • Take an easy walk and do some stretching.

✳ Squat Strikes

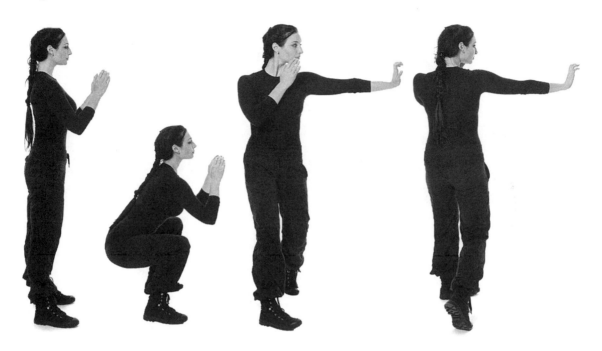

Primary Fitness Target • Glutes

Primary Self-Defense Target • Attacker's eyes

Starting Position • Off-Guard Stance

Movement • Full Squat | Combatives

Movement 1: Complete a full Squat (reference the Fitness Placement Test in Chapter 8 if needed).

Movement 2: When you return to Off-Guard Stance, tuck in your pelvis for the full range of motion and complete two Palm Strikes. Those at the intermediate level will follow with an Elbow Combative—or if you're at an advanced level, perform any three combatives you like. Remember: technique over speed. Twist and pivot on the ball of your foot through the combatives to get the full range of motion. This is a great way of conditioning your reaction when you need to defend from a neutral stance against a threat—plus you get an extra contraction of your core and glute muscles!

Beginner • 12 Squats with Palm Strikes

Intermediate • 12 Squats with 2 Palm Strikes, 2 Elbow Combatives

Advanced • 12 Squats with any 3 upper-body combatives

Advanced Plus • 12 to 15 Squats with any 3 upper-body combatives

EXERCISE 2

✱ Forward Lunge Combatives

Primary Fitness Target • Glutes

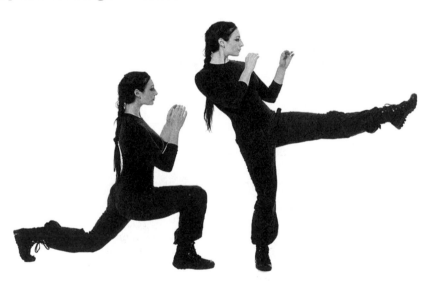

Primary Self-Defense Target • Advancing into your ranges

Starting Position • Standing with feet together

Movement • Deep Front Lunge, Front Push Kick, and Front Elbow

   Movement 1: Take a deep step forward and lower your hips to complete a full Lunge.

   Movement 2: Transition forward so that your rear foot takes a step into Survival

Stance. Immediately engage in a Front Push Kick (reference Chapter 6 if needed). Remember to push your hips forward to achieve the full range of motion, optimal force, and contraction of your core and glutes.

Movement 3: Before your front foot comes down, engage in a near-side Horizontal Elbow and make sure to achieve the full range of motion by completing a full twist.

Beginner • 12 Lunges | 12 Push Kicks

Intermediate • 12 Lunges | 12 Push Kicks and Elbows

Advanced • 12 to 15 Lunges, Push Kicks, and Elbows (continuous)

Advanced Plus • 12 to 15 Lunges and individual continuous combative combinations

---

EXERCISE 3

✸ Tricep Kicking Get-Ups

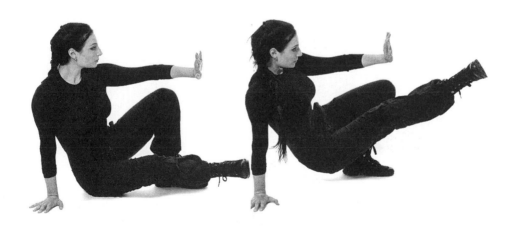

Primary Fitness Target • Full body

Primary Self-Defense Targets • Knee, face—and practicing the fundamentals of rape defense, in particular by practicing a Push Kick as you transition from ground range to standing up

Starting Position • Sit-Up Defensive Position. This is the defensive position you can adopt when transitioning from your back to standing up in your full Survival Stance. As you are in a seated position, support yourself by placing one hand behind you, and keeping your other hand in a defensive guard position. When it comes to your legs, place one foot flat on the ground so that your knee is close to your chest as your other leg is slightly bent and raised in front of you with the heel flexed—ready to kick if needed.

Movement • Continuous Kicks from Ground

Movement 1: Engage in a Push Kick, using your heel to target an attacker's knee or face. Make sure to raise your hips during every kick. Meanwhile, use your nearside arm to ward off the attacker.

Movement 2: Immediately return the leg to starting position and repeat on the other side. Try changing up your visualized target from the attacker's knees to the groin and face.

Beginner • 8 Tricep Push Kicks

Intermediate • 15 Tricep Push Kicks

Advanced • 8 Tricep Push Kicks with full Get-Up (see page 129)

Advanced Plus • 12 Tricep Push Kicks with full Get-Up

EXERCISE 4

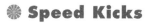 **Speed Kicks**

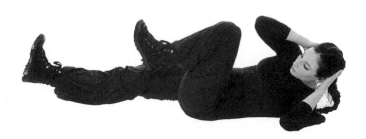

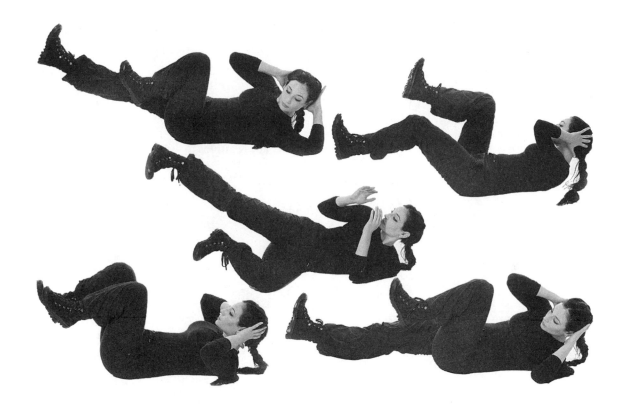

Primary Fitness Target • Core

Primary Self-Defense Targets • Explosive kicks to available targets on an attacker—this is especially effective against an attacker who is standing over you

Starting Position • Survival Ground Stance, with both knees tucked into the chest

Movement • Continuous Kick from Ground

Movement 1: Tuck your chest to your knees to engage your core. Maintain your guarded upper body position and core contraction throughout the entire duration of the exercise.

Movement 2: Extend one heel out as you redirect that same side arm diagonally away.

Movement 3: Return your kicking leg to the starting position as you extend the other leg. At this point, you will continue through movements 2 and 3 until you have completed your repetitions for the set.

Beginner • 10 to 15 Speed Kicks

Intermediate • 20 to 30 Speed Kicks

Advanced • 20 Speed Kicks at all angles. To apply your kick at all angles, make sure to envision different targets at different heights to help you tighten your core from a variety of angles, as you practice a real application of kicking someone.

Advanced Plus • 30 to 40 Speed Kicks at all angles

EXERCISE 5

❋ Brace Crunches

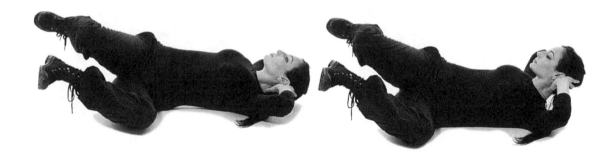

Primary Fitness Target • Core

Primary Self-Defense Target • Practicing rape defense fundamentals, in particular the ground survival position and bracing your legs to prevent an attacker from getting in between your legs

Starting Position • Brace position. The Brace position is the defensive position on the ground that will ensure you are able to prevent an attacker from further advancing his body in between your legs. The Brace position means that you are on your back, with both feet flexed and one leg "bracing" across your body's center line, simply by driving that leg's shin bone across the attacker's hips, as your other heel is placed on the imaginary shin bone of the attacker. As you establish this defensive position with your legs, simply raise your arms to place your hands as if they were in the Survival Stance to complete your defensive protection for your whole body.

Movement • Brace Crunches

Movement: From Brace position, place both hands behind your head, flare your elbows outward, and lift your chest to the ceiling to complete one crunch.

Beginner • 15 Brace Crunches

Intermediate • 30 Brace Crunches

Advanced • 45 Brace Crunches

Advanced Plus • 60 Brace Crunches

BURNOUT VARIATION

❋ Defensive Jumping Jacks

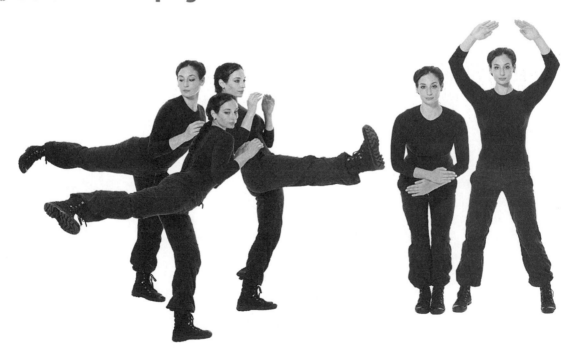

This is a great variation to your burnout rounds. It will keep your heart rate up and force you to condition your kicks from a more difficult starting position. Remember, fight for your technique! Starting from a neutral stance, complete a Push Kick Side Kick, and Rear Kick and then return to neutral stance and do a jumping jack. Repeat on fast speed for 1 minute.

Cardio Combative Challenge

For Weeks 3 and 4, do a series of continuous combatives to your favorite music. Perform as many rounds as possible of a chosen series of combatives without compromising your technique. I want you to choose a basic combination that you would like to improve or to create a new combination. For example, one combo you might try is Near Snap Kick, Near Palm Strike, Rear Palm Strike, Rear Snap Kick, New Near Fist Strike, Defensive Knee, and Sky Elbow. The options are endless!

WEEKS 5 AND 6 WORKOUTS

Great job on getting this far! It's been a month, and I can promise you that you're already much stronger than you were before. Now we're entering the final phase of the *Weapons of Fitness* workout. Please fill your training schedule below.

SCHEDULE TRACKER							
Day of Week	Day 1	Day 2	Day 3	Day 4	Day 5	Day 6	Day 7
Weapons of Fitness							
Cardio Combatives							
Soteria Pyramid Minutes							
Visualization Minutes							
Nutrition							
Inner Soteria							

SCHEDULE TRACKER							
Day of Week	Day 1	Day 2	Day 3	Day 4	Day 5	Day 6	Day 7
Weapons of Fitness							
Cardio Combatives							
Soteria Pyramid Minutes							
Visualization Minutes							
Nutrition							
Inner Soteria							

WEAPONS OF FITNESS WEEKS 5 AND 6						
Exercise	Beginner	Intermediate	Advanced	Advanced +	Burnouts	Sets/Reps
Warm-Up						
Ground Push Kicks	8 Pelvis Tilts	10 Ground Push Kicks	15 Ground Push Kicks	20 Ground Push Kicks	30–60 seconds of alternating combatives OR Jumping Jacks OR Skips	3 Sets
Direct Elbow Corner Kicks	10 Direct Elbows | 10 Kicks	15 Direct Elbow | 15 Kicks	20 Direct Elbows and Kicks (continuous)	25 Direct Elbows and Kicks (continuous)		
Rear Lunge Elbow Kick	10 Lunges | 10 Swinging Rear Elbows	10 Lunges into Swinging Elbows	10 Lunges into Swinging Elbows	10 Lunges, Swinging Elbows, and Rear Kicks		
Combat Plank and Ground Side Kick	5 Ground Side Kicks | 20-second Side Plank	10 Ground Side Kicks | 20-second Side Plank	10 Ground Side Kicks | 45-second Side Plank	12 Ground Side Kicks | 60-second Side Plank		
Striking Sit-Ups	12 Sit-Ups with Palm Strikes	12 Sit-Ups with Elbow Strikes	15 Sit-Ups with Palm Strikes and Elbow Strikes	25 Sit-Ups with any combative combination		
Cooldown and Stretch						

WEAPONS OF FITNESS WORKOUT BREAKDOWN

Warm-Up • Warm up with dynamic stretches and combatives according to the instructions on pages 136–139.

Exercises • Do 3 sets of repetitions or timed durations for each exercise, making sure each set is followed by 1 minute of burnouts

Cooldown • Take an easy walk and do some stretching.

EXERCISE 1

❋ Ground Push Kicks

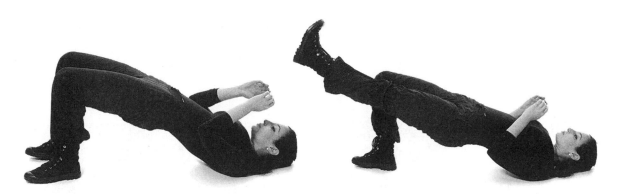

Primary Fitness Target • Glutes

Primary Self-Defense Targets • Knee, groin, face

Starting Position • Lie on your back and bend your knees so that your feet are flat on the ground. Raise your arms to cover your face as you do in Survival Stance.

Movement • Pelvis Tilt with a simultaneous Push Kick

Movement 1: Dig your heels into the ground, and as you raise your pelvis to the ceiling, bring one knee into your chest and prepare that leg to do a Push Kick.

Movement 2: Extend the heel or ball of the foot into an imaginary target. Remember that the Push Kick is aimed at the attacker's knee, groin, or face; visualize different targets as you work your way through the sets.

Beginner • 8 Pelvis Tilts—Work on building power for a Push Kick by focusing only on the pelvis tilt, which is the source of the kick's power

Intermediate • 10 Ground Push Kicks

Advanced • 15 Ground Push Kicks

Advanced Plus • 20 Ground Push Kicks

Direct Elbow Corner Kicks

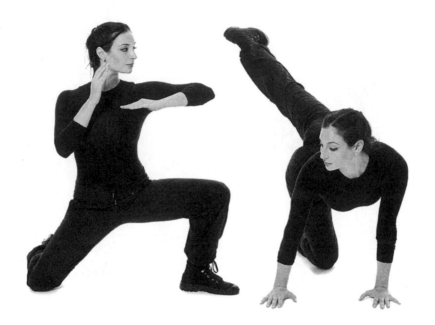

Primary Fitness Targets • Glutes, core

Primary Self-Defense Target • Working on range of motion for combatives

Starting Position • On your knees with your arms in the Survival Stance position

Movement • Side Lunge with Direct Elbow into Corner Kick

Movement 1: Take a deep step to the side and simultaneously engage in a Direct Side Elbow.

Movement 2: Immediately transition to all fours and extend your leg out so that you drive the heel to the rear cross corner. Remember to keep your chest up throughout the whole movement.

Beginner • 10 Direct Elbows | 10 Kicks

Intermediate • 15 Direct Elbows | 15 Kicks

Advanced • 20 Direct Elbows and Kicks (continuous)

Advanced Plus • 25 Direct Elbows and Kicks (continuous)

EXERCISE 3

�֍ Rear Lunge Combatives

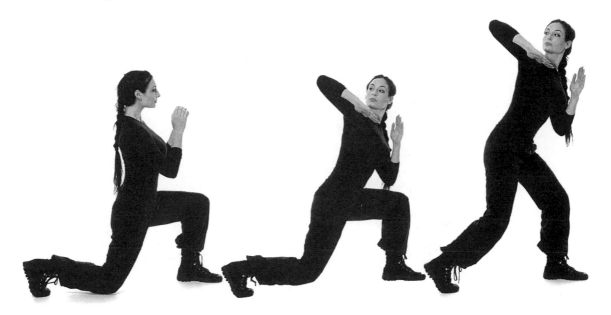

Primary Fitness Target • Glutes

Primary Self-Defense Targets • Face, groin

Starting Position • Off-Guard Stance

Movement • Rear Lunge and Rear Elbow | Rear Kick

Movement 1: Take a deep step to the back and drop your hips into a full lunge.

Movement 2: From your lunge position, complete 1 Swinging Rear Elbow. Beginners can first raise your hips by straightening your legs before you complete the Rear Swinging Elbow.

Movement 3: Bring both feet together for a split second and immediately do a Rear Kick.

Beginner • 10 Lunges and 10 Swinging Rear Elbows—You can first raise your hips to straighten your legs before you do the Elbows.

Intermediate • 10 Lunges and 10 Swinging Elbows, executed when you have returned from the lunge

Advanced • 10 Lunges and 10 Swinging Elbows, executed at the lowest level of the lunge

Advanced Plus • 10 Lunges, 10 Swinging Elbows, and 10 Rear Kicks—Visualize a rear target for using your Swinging Rear Elbow and a rear target for the Rear Kick, as if you are facing multiple attackers or are facing a new angle against an attacker.

✳ Combat Plank and Ground Side Kick

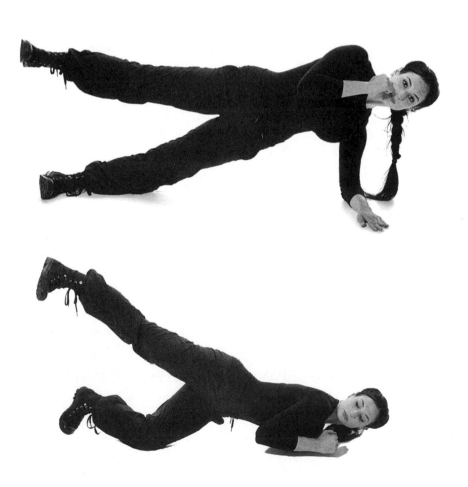

Primary Fitness Targets • Glutes, core

Primary Self-Defense Target • Side kick to the knee

Starting Position • Side lean. Starting on the ground, lie down on your side so that you are resting on your shoulder. Make sure both arms are in Survival Position.

Movement • Raising your hips while simultaneously extending your heel

Movement 1: First spot your target (the attacker's knee) when you are in your starting position. As you raise your hips, bring your kicking knee into your chest. Then extend the heel of your kicking foot outward to make contact with the attacker. Make sure that you cross-rotate your upper body so that your right hip rotates inward and is at a 45-degree angle with the ground.

Movement 2: Hold a static Side Plank and raise one arm in front of you as you would if you were in Survival Stance

Beginner • 5 Ground Side Kicks followed by a 20-second Side Plank

Intermediate • 10 Ground Side Kicks followed by a 20-second Side Plank

Advanced • 10 Ground Side Kicks followed by a 45-second Side Plank

Advanced Plus • 12 Ground Side Kicks followed by a 60-second Side Plank
Remember to complete the sets on both sides.

EXERCISE 5

✳ Striking Sit-Ups

Primary Fitness Target • Core

Primary Self-Defense Target • Face

Starting Position • Lie on your back with your knees bent, your feet flat on the ground and your arms up to guard your face.

Movement • Full Sit-Up with a combative strike

Movement 1: Do a full Sit-Up by raising your chest to the ceiling.

Movement 2: When you have completed the full Sit-Up, engage in two upper-body combatives before returning to the starting position.

Beginner • 12 Sit-Ups with Palm Strikes

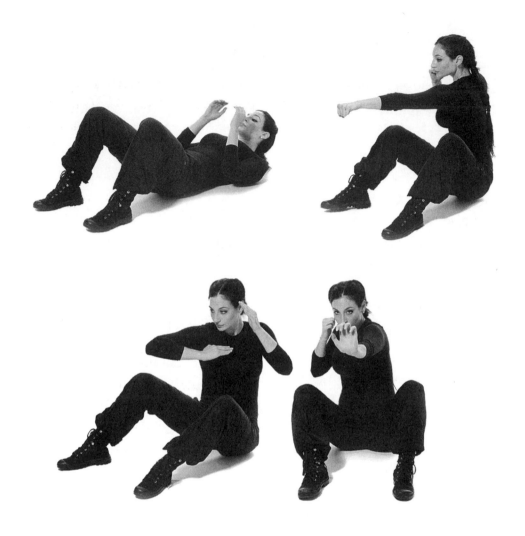

Intermediate • 12 Sit-Ups with Elbow Strikes

Advanced • 15 Sit-Ups with Palm Strikes and Elbow Strikes

Advanced Plus • 25 Sit-Ups with any combative combination

Cardio Combative Challenges

For Weeks 5 and 6, your cardio routine again consists of doing a series of continuous combatives to your favorite music. Pick a continuous combative flow and perform as many rounds as possible without compromising your technique.

Bonus Workout

Before you continue, I wanted to provide you with a bonus workout that introduces you to one of my Full Defense Workouts. A Full Defense Workout includes a certain progression of exercises that are based on specific steps needed to be accomplished in a Soteria Method defense. For this bonus workout, I am going to show you how to practice the featured Ground Survival defense in a full body workout.

Starting Position: On the ground on your back (i.e., in the ground range that you're trying to avoid being caught in).

Exercise 1: Brace Crunches: This is to ensure that you can create a "gate" against your attacker's attempt to get in between your legs.

Exercise 2: Ground Push Kicks: Once you create the Brace, immediately engage in a Ground Push Kick to disrupt your attacker's thought process and to push both his head and body backward.

Exercise 3: Tricep Push Kicks: Once you complete the first kick, you want to transition back up to your feet. However, you must always be prepared to engage in another kick, which is why I want you to practice another Push Kick from an upright seated position.

Exercise 4: Self-Defense Get-Up: Practice getting up safely once you have created the opening and opportunity to do so.

Exercise 5: Full Ground Survival Defense: That is right! For the final exercise, you will go through exercises 1 through 4 in a single repetition progression to practice the full defense as you would against a real attacker. This is a great challenge because from an overall toning and conditioning perspective, you will be forcing your body to recruit and contract muscles in a whole new way.

When you are completing my Full Defense Workouts, make sure that you challenge yourself to maintain technical excellence and consistency as you place your mental focus on visualizing yourself applying the moves against an imaginary attacker.

IMPROVISED WEAPON
BONUS WORKOUT

If you should ever face violence, objects in your immediate vicinity could help you defend yourself. Are you carrying keys? Those are basically miniature daggers. Do you have an umbrella? That will function just fine as a makeshift bat. Is there a chair nearby? It can serve as a shield and is very tough for an attacker to circumvent. I want you to start thinking creatively about your surroundings. Here are some of my favorite improvised weapons, along with exercises to help you train and get comfortable using them.

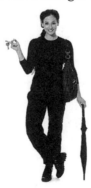

CHAIR

A chair is a great improvised weapon and can serve as a shield around your torso.

✸ **Chair Swings**

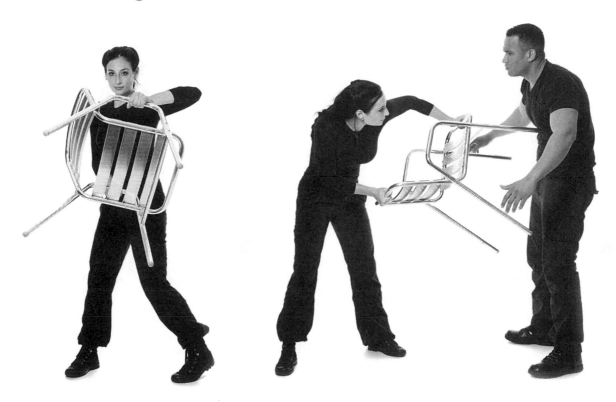

If you swing a chair in a figure-eight motion, it is like having additional arms of steel with which to strike your attacker. Swinging the chair in a figure-eight motion as you simultaneously extend and pull the chair from your body will give you a great alternative to the burnouts you've been doing. The added weight of the chair will help give your muscles endurance and tone.

✳ Chair Lunges

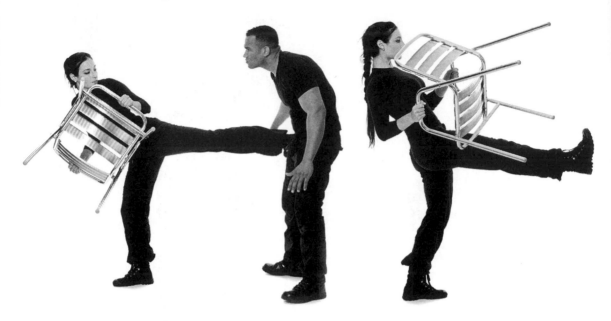

Adding in Front and Side Kicks when using a chair as either a shield or a weapon is extremely effective when defending against both armed and unarmed attacks. This exercise is a great way to get comfortable doing lower-body combatives with an improvised weapon.

Movement 1 • Lunge

Beginner/Intermediate • Feel free to use the chair as a bar to help you keep your balance from a full lunge into a Front or Side Kick.

Advanced/Advanced Plus • While holding the chair, engage in a full lunge

Movement 2 • Engage in Combatives

Beginner/Intermediate • While using the chair as a bar, return from your lunge and immediately use your rear leg to do a Push Kick

Advanced/Advanced Plus • While holding the chair and returning from your lunge, immediately engage in either a Front or a Side Kick. Feel free to add on chair swings as part of each repetition.

PURSE

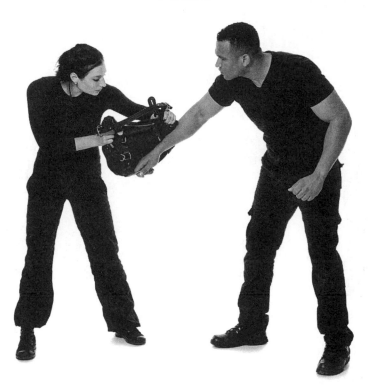

My purse is one of my favorite improvised weapons and shields. It is great to use for redirecting an active knife attack, stopping a hook punch, and hitting someone with. I always hold my purse around my arm and across my stomach to avoid theft and also so it protects me and is readily available.

✳ Purse Crunches and Sit-Ups

When I need to add more weight into my exercises, I love to bring in heavier improvised weapons, in addition to working with classic fitness equipment such as free weights. This simply gets me more comfortable with unknown objects and conditions my mind for how I would use them while completing my reps. Try my

Purse Crunches and Sit-Ups and fill up your purse with as much as you want to adjust the weight!

Movement • Complete a full Crunch or Sit-Up

Beginner/Intermediate • As many Purse Crunches as you can do in 1 minute

Advanced/Advanced Plus • Up to 60 Purse Sit-Ups per set

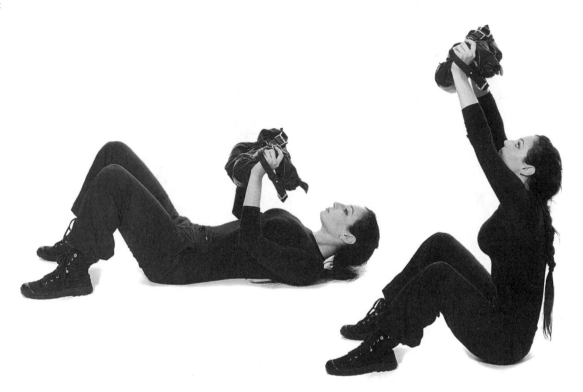

UMBRELLA

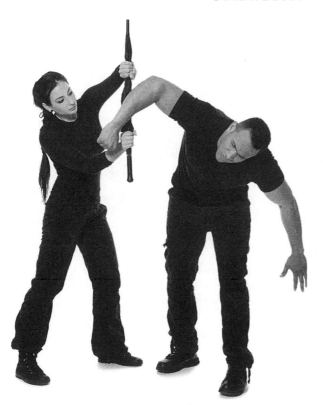 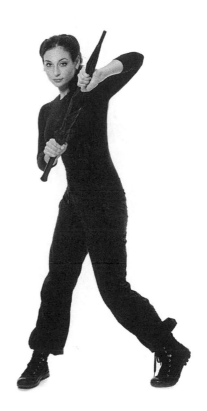

The umbrella is a great impact weapon and falls close to the structure of a bat or stick. You can use it as a shield against a knife attack, swing it as a weapon, and integrate it into your combatives to hit vulnerable areas on an attacker, such as his neck and knees.

❋ Umbrella Squats

These moves are a great way to practice and get inspired by the umbrella's potential blocking and swinging impacts.

Movement • Starting with your hand on either end of the umbrella, complete a full squat. As you drop your hips, extend your arms out.

Beginner/Intermediate • Perform as many squats as you can in 1 minute.

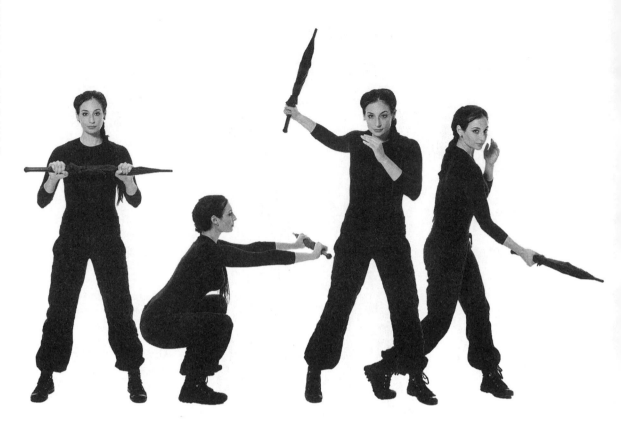

Advanced/Advanced Plus • Perform a squat, and when you return to starting position, immediately go into a block position with your umbrella. Then attempt to engage in a Push Kick and defensive swings immediately after to end the repetition. Do as many reps as you can in 1 minute.

IMPACT WEAPON

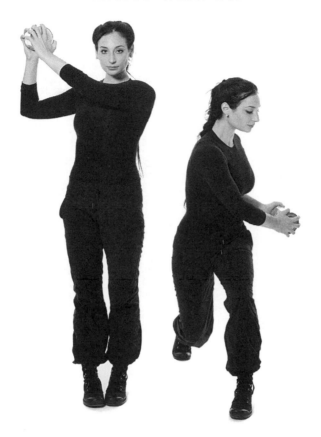

In the image above, I am using a heavy paint can as an improvised impact weapon. This can easily be replaced with a snow globe or a piece of home decor. I recommend having certain fixtures placed at certain positions into your home, dorm room, or office in case you need to gain access to something to defend yourself with immediately.

✺ Impact Hammer

Movement • As you go into a full lunge, swing an improvised impact weapon across your body. Return to the starting position.

All Levels • Perform as many reps as you can in 1 minute.

KEYS

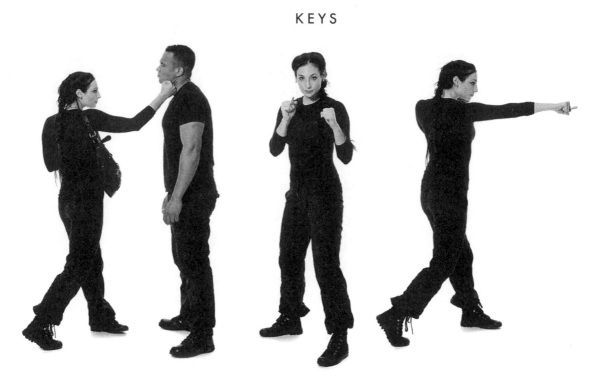

Your keys are a great weapon to use in a close-range attack. I consider this a convenient improvised weapon because you tend to always have your keys on you—especially when in potentially dangerous situations like inside a parking lot or garage or walking home and up your driveway to your door. I recommend buying a large, strong key, and while you're walking around, placing it between your first and second finger, angled out like a dagger.

✺ Key Burnouts

I like to bring my keys into my burnout rounds to try to practice different angles.

Movement • While holding your keys like a weapon, perform alternating upper-body combatives.

All Levels • Perform as many repetitions as you can within 1 minute. Remember not to compromise technique for speed.

PROTECTING YOUR LIFE

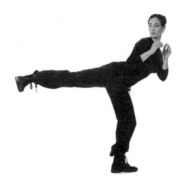

CREATING AND PROTECTING A LIFE YOU LOVE

Attack Life. Don't Let Life Attack You" has become my mantra—my road map to creating my best life. All of my personal discoveries that have led me to reclaiming my life have been put in the Soteria Method for you. I discovered the positives in self-defense, and it changed every aspect of my life. In this chapter, I'll review what we've covered and show you what I know self-defense can do for you.

I asked you in the beginning of this book to give me your word that you would stick to this plan and be open to the possibility of a new perspective on life. Your word is everything, and when you commit yourself to a new opportunity, you must surrender all preconceptions and persevere through any negative reactions or feelings in order to give that opportunity or perspective the attention it needs. Take a moment now to remind yourself of what you have already accomplished through keeping your word and reading this book. Continue to commit to remaining open to new possibilities, free of judgment or bias—and watch your life's potential unfold.

You can adopt a lifestyle full of safety habits that will remove you from the path of danger and help prevent violence. Here are my top tips for violence prevention and safety, which you can immediately implement.

MY TOP VIOLENCE PREVENTION AND SAFETY TIPS

Here's how you can make yourself a hard target by increasing your situational awareness (your understanding of your surroundings).

1 *Use Peripheral Vision:* Use your peripheral vision when in public so that you are automatically seeing more and will therefore recognize something out of place sooner.

2 *Know Where You Are Going:* When you know your destination and how to get there, you will avoid getting caught in the wrong area—and you will also portray a sense of alertness that will make you a harder target.

3 *Cut the Distractions:* When you are traveling, eliminate any distractions, such as listening to music or texting on your phone, that will lower your awareness of your environment and make you an easy target who can be caught off guard.

4 *Use Technology:* Always have your devices charged, and use a map or GPS app on your phone so that as you go from place to place, you have a clear understanding of where you are and what is nearby—and you have a fully charged phone for communication.

5 *Identify Real Exits:* Where is your exit if you need one? Remember, *real* exits are ones that immediately lead to a safe location.

6 *Trust Your Intuition:* Trust your gut when it sets off an alarm that someone has crossed into your public and personal circles.

7 *Use Barriers and Surface Areas:* All surface areas can be used to your advantage. You can eliminate a threat or an act of violence from directly behind you by standing in front of a wall or a pillar (this will keep someone from creeping up behind you or sucker punching you from the back). Any piece of furniture or barrier-like object can be used to keep distance between you and an attacker—or can just get in your way. Be smart with your surroundings.

8 *Carry a Purse:* Not only is the purse a great improvised weapon, but also you should always carry with you keys, extra cash, forms of ID, a charger, and a pen (improvised weapon).

9 *Use Improvised Weapons:* Get in the practice of locating improvised weapons around you. Remember, anything can be used as an improvised weapon when your objective is to disrupt the attacker's thought process.

10 *Eliminate Predictability:* The best routine is no routine. Don't make yourself predictable, even if you do have a regular schedule. Whether this means taking a different route home, or waiting with people and taking a safe ride home, it all adds up to making you a harder target to anticipate.

11 *Buddy Up:* Whether you are working out, going out on a date, or attending a college party, make sure you have a safety buddy or someone who can help keep an eye out for you. At the very least, make sure someone you trust knows where you are.

12 *Scan for Weapons:* If you do see a suspicious person, immediately scan his hands for a weapon. Take note of any other obvious signs of aggression through body language and verbal language.

13 *Confirm a Threat:* Once you have scanned the suspicious person, if you can escape, that should be your first defense. However, if you can't escape, you will be faced either with an active attack, which means that the attacker is on the move toward you, or with a nonactive threat, which means that you have identified and confirmed the threat but he is not yet active. These scenarios are what you can begin to train in your visualization minutes.

14 *Find Safe Locations:* Identify locations that can offer you immediate safety, such as a crowded street, a coffee shop with people inside, or any other professional establishment such as a bank, police station, or office building. I recommend knowing safe locations on routes that you frequent, and if you're traveling somewhere new, do some research on the Internet beforehand.

15 *Visualize How You Would React to a Violent Threat:* Again, nothing will be retained if you don't train for reality. It is best to play out the possibilities in your mind and visualize your reaction so that you can get your survival mindset familiar with the available options and necessary survival tactics.

No matter how safely you live your life, you can still be targeted for violence, anywhere, anytime, and for any reason—which is why you are taking control of your own safety right now.

Now, let's go back through the tactics you learned in this book and look at how you can apply them in your everyday life.

RACE REACTION MODEL
Self-Defense Application

Understand that your mind has to progress through four reactive cognitive phases against the threat or act of violence. These are recognizing, analyzing, composing, and executing (RACE) a defense. Every second spent training is crucial to building a foundation based on accurate and timely reactions.

Life Application

You don't have to settle for your first reaction to a negative situation. You don't need to settle and fall under the rule of negative thoughts or feelings associated with fears, anxiety, doubt, or any other insecurities. You can and will train yourself to react to threats in real time, with real solutions.

NO RULES
Self-Defense Application

The difference between self-defense and some other martial arts is that self-defense has no rules. This allows you to utilize your survival mindset to do whatever it takes to defend yourself.

Life Application

Don't live your life by rules or limitations that hold you back from going after your own self-protection and achieving your dreams.

3-FACTOR COMBATIVE THEORY

Self-Defense Application

So you can build the right form and technique, I have outlined three factors, or reference points, that have to be met during each repetition:

1. *Target:* The top targets are the eyes, face, and groin.
2. *Surface Area:* The body part you strike with should be the strongest and least fragile surface area.
3. *Range of Motion:* Train for a consistent range of motion. Use the Combative Twist or the Hip Thrust to help gain consistency.

Life Application

1. *Target:* What is it that you want out of life, and what do you need to target to create the life or moments you want to experience?
2. *Surface Area:* What are the skills, talents, and passions that will allow you to actualize that dream?
3. *Range of Motion:* How far are you willing to go to turn your dreams into reality?

STRIKING THROUGH THE TARGET

Self-Defense Application

We want to aim to strike through the target so that the attacker receives the full amount of force. Training to strike through the attacker means that you will need to know your personal ranges and what combatives fall under what range. The four ranges are long range, medium range, control range, and ground range.

Life Application

Don't just do the minimum; give everything your all. Let your ability hit through each target you want to achieve in every aspect of your life—and see how new possibilities present themselves to you. One of my greatest fears is looking back down the road and knowing that I didn't give everything my all. You have one life, and you need to squeeze *everything* you want out of it!

MUSCLE MEMORY

Self-Defense Application

You need to build muscle memory to stay within the composition phase so that you can continually react to the threat, instead of focusing on technical execution. Here's the equation for building muscle memory: MUSCLE MEMORY = MINDFULNESS + FORM + CONSISTENCY

Life Application

The one thing you can train consistently is keeping your word. Be mindful of your commitments, see through what you have committed to, and be consistent—don't fall for an excuse or a justification. Doing the right thing and being dependable will allow you to move forward in a positive direction.

SOTERIA METHOD SURVIVAL PYRAMID

Self-Defense Application

Stop: Stop the initial threat and escape if you can. If you cannot, then . . .

Secure: Close in and secure the attacker's arm or body. Remember, you will have this temporarily, so you will need to . . .

Strike: Continue to disrupt his thought process and structure until you can . . .

Survive: Neutralize or safely escape the situation

Life Application

Stop: Block negative influences or energies from impacting your life.

Secure: Take the time to secure your future—your personal safety, your health, your dreams.

Strike: Reach out and go for your goals. Taking action is the best way to get to where you want to go.

Survive: No matter what challenges you may face, there will be a way to move forward—by using positivity as your weapon.

THE POSITIVE ANGLE APPROACH
Self-Defense Application

Training to find the positive in the situation will help you break through the mental and physical freezes when switching into that tactical survival mindset.

Life Application

You can train to find the positive in any situation. It will be difficult, but you will start to feel and see the beauty and growth that comes when you keep on persevering.

SURVIVAL MINDSET
Self-Defense Application

Operate with a mindset that has the single objective of surviving a threat or an attack—at all costs.

Life Application

Your survival mindset for life should be your wanting to survive and overcome any challenges as you attack and create the life you want. I constantly found myself applying my survival mindset to get through all my personal and professional challenges—as I felt that I was able to apply these tools against any negativity and conflict while concentrating on the positives in my life.

No matter what trauma you face, you can always overcome it in a positive and meaningful way. You must find a cause, one even greater than yourself, that will allow you to concentrate your energy on making important gains or changes in your life. This could be a person, moment, or tangible object, as long as it resonates deeply and personally with you.

PERSONAL BOUNDARIES
Self-Defense Application

As you build an authentic survival mindset, you will be forced to break through mental and physical boundaries to overcome the mental and physical freezes that take place in your RACE Reaction to a threat or an act of violence.

Life Application

We all have emotional, psychological, and mental boundaries—some obvious and others not so obvious to ourselves. However, in order to grow and explore new possibilities, we must push against these boundaries and work our way through the roadblocks that are holding us back from seeing what life has to offer.

COMBATIVE OBJECTIVE
Self-Defense Application

Your objective is to disrupt the attacker's thought process to buy yourself time to make your next move. Don't just rely on a series of moves and hope for the best or hope for an outcome or result that you cannot control. Disrupt an attacker's thought process and use this to your advantage.

Life Application

Don't place importance on factors outside your control. As in the self-defense application, you cannot guarantee any certain reaction from your attacker, and you cannot guarantee any certain reaction out of life. Prepare to adapt—as that is your greatest strategy for survival—and focus on what you can achieve.

USE OF FORCE

Self-Defense Application

You are allowed to use only as much force as the amount of force that is used on you.

Life Application

If someone or a situation attacks you with aggression or with the intention to bring you down, raise your own bar to protect yourself. Be aware of the variables of your situation and react accordingly with an aim to remove yourself from this threatening situation.

KEEP AN EYE ON THE ATTACKER

Self-Defense Application

I always say that you should always have at least one eye on your attacker, no matter what, so that you can visually take in any changing dynamics or variables. This concept helps you achieve the related goal of never giving your attacker your back.

Life Application

Always keep an eye on your potential, nothing else. Don't worry about what the competition is doing or what you are not doing. Focus on what needs to be done so you can be your best, and you will see how far you go. If you are looking sideways or behind you, opportunities may be missed.

SIMPLICITY IS SURVIVAL
Self-Defense Application

The running theme here is simplicity when it comes to self-defense. You won't always have the ability to think deeply on how to react when confronted with a violent threat or an attack. It is with this understanding that we must simplify self-defense, and I have done that for you with my Soteria Method Survival Pyramid. I have stripped down what you need to know, what you need to train, and what you need to visualize to get your mind and body working together.

Life Application

Find success in the simple things in life and you will see that happiness is all around you. Happiness comes from finding a common peace with who you are and what you can do for the world. Try to simplify every aspect of your life, without making excuses not to do certain things. Fight for the simplicity in each day to find authentic happiness in every aspect of your life.

YOUR BEAUTY
Fitness Application

When I made the decision to stop judging my body based on pounds, measurements, or how "cut" I was from one day to another, I began to appreciate the natural curves of my body and saw that my body became its best when I mentally let go of this image of "perfection." My body is perfect—because I am alive and it allows me do what I need to. I refuse to let any perceived shortcoming in some arbitrary measurement define how beautiful I am.

Life Application

I realize that it's hard not to judge yourself against the norms of beauty portrayed by society and the media. But this is one of the battles that we as women must face and engage in so that we protect how we feel about ourselves—and ultimately protect how much we can enjoy every moment. When I finally began to look inside to find what made me feel happy and what brought beauty into my life, I ultimately found my inner feminine strength to live my life my way.

VISUALIZATION (MOST IMPORTANT)

You need to visualize practicing your self-defense concepts and tactics in real-life scenarios so that you can create fake "real experiences" for your mind to draw on when composing a defense against the threat or act of violence. Visualizing is my biggest secret to personal success and to finding happiness, purpose, and a new form of strength to apply to every aspect of my life. I used this ability to visualize the world that I wanted to live in, the moments that I would dedicate myself to living, and the possibility of getting everything I want out of life.

CONCLUSION

I want you to use this book as a way to transform physically and mentally into your own warrior goddess and to protect the life you deserve to live.

The breakthroughs that I have achieved are what led me on this path of self-discovery and resulted in the creation of the Soteria Method, which I have introduced to you in this book—your guide to reclaiming your life for *you!*

As you continue to apply the *Weapons of Fitness* workouts in your life, you will start to see how simple the Soteria Method is when it comes to self-defense. I want you to apply the lifesaving concepts that I discovered, in addition to your own discoveries, as you embrace the Soteria in you. I want you to wake up and knock out your fears. I want you to prepare for moments of weakness by arming yourself with your dreams for a better life and a more authentic you. I want you to find what you are thankful for and what you can do each day to make the world a better place. I want you to get tactical in making your dreams a reality, and I want you to fight to protect the life you are creating. And finally, I want you to breathe and let your emotional guard down, knowing that you are taking your safety into your own hands and mind—as no one has the power to change what you see, what you feel, or how you react to life. You have only one life. Now create it, live it, love it, and protect it!

INDEX

abdominals
  combatives and, 55, 98
  of Zeisler, 3
active attacks, static vs., 106
  Adam's apple, 111
  adaptive mindset, 47
  aerobics, 142, 145–46
  aggressors, aggression, 14, 203
  combatives and, 142
  force and, 209
  RACE Reaction Model and, 18
  self-defense and, 130
  stances and, 45
  survival mindset and, 20–21
alcohol, 102–3, 147
analyzing
  RACE Reaction Model and,
      17–20, 106, 204
  self-defense and, 106
  survival mindset and, 20
angles
  Angled Arm Extensions, 67
  Angled Hammer Fists, 61, 63
  Angle Elbows, 72

breaking the angle, 44–45, 131
  combatives and, 61, 63, 65–68,
      70, 72, 75, 80, 83, 86,
      95
  positive-angle approach and,
      33–34, 65, 121, 207
  Rear Angle Elbow Combatives,
      72
  self-defense and, 7, 113–15, 131,
      207
  stances and, 33–34, 36–38,
      44–45
  workouts and, 144, 169, 178
ankles
  combatives and, 53
  workouts and, 136, 139, 169
arms, 14, 26
  Angled Arm Extensions, 67
  combatives and, 52–53, 55,
      62–63, 65, 67–69, 78, 80,
      86, 91, 97
  positive-angle approach and, 34
  self-defense and, 106–8, 113–14,
      116–19, 122–23, 125

stances and, 36, 38
  workouts and, 136–37, 139, 154,
      164, 166, 176–78, 183–84,
      187, 191, 195
attackers
  keeping eye on, 209
  multiple, 98, 105–6, 186

back, 209. *See also* rear, rear side
  Back Hammer Fists, 7, 61,
      64–65, 117–18
  combatives and, 85–87, 98
  self-defense and, 117, 120
  workouts and, 155, 168, 170,
      183, 187, 189
balance
  combatives and, 83
  self-defense and, 108, 119
  stances and, 36, 38–39, 43, 108,
      119
  workouts and, 152, 192
barriers, 58, 86, 202
bats, 106, 190

215